DR. SEBI CURE FOR ACNE

The Complete Step-by-Step Guide on How to Cure
Acne Naturally in Less Than 1-Week and Prevent
Relapse. Includes 7-Day Alkaline Diet Plan to
Rebalance pH Levels

Table of Contents

Introduction

Acne is a skin burden that may be unpleasant and distressing, whether it develops during your adolescence or later in life. It can often feel like an arduous struggle against the breakouts, from pus-filled pimples to their lingering scars. However, don't get the blemish blues. The first step toward cleaner skin is understanding what causes these breakouts and learning about essential components that can help minimize their appearance, intensity, and spread.

Acne is the most prevalent skin condition in the United States, affecting up to 90% of teenagers at some time. Acne can have serious psychological and social consequences that are difficult to assess. Acne, if left untreated, can cause substantial and long-term skin damage. Acne is a complex condition, which makes it tough to treat.

There are four key variables that contribute to acne:

- Hormonal imbalances and excessive oil production
- Colonization of Propionibacterium (bacteria levels increase with excess oil production).
- Inflammation.
- A typical or disorganized shedding of skin cells from the skin's surface.

To treat acne as successfully as possible, the treatment strategy should target all four causes.

Hormonal problems in women can be addressed with oral contraceptives and sometimes with a drug called spironolactone (more often used in adult-onset acne), and both of these will usually lower oil production. For males, the only option to minimize oil production is to use Accutane, which is only recommended for severe acne, especially if the acne is causing disfiguring scars.

Bacteria can be treated with prescription medicines in both topical and oral forms. Topically, there are antibiotic preparations (such as clindamycin) and medicines that are not antibiotics but have antibiotic characteristics, such as benzoyl peroxide. If feasible, oral antibiotics should be low-dose and slow-release. Because they have anti-inflammatory effects, -cyclin antibiotics such as minocycline, doxycycline, or tetracycline are often utilized. There is a prescription-only, low-dose, slow-release version of doxycycline that is safer for long-term usage. Inflammation is a severe condition that is sometimes overlooked. Certain people are more pro-inflammatory than others, making them more prone to cysts, nodules, redness, and pustular lesions associated with severe acne. Topical and oral anti-inflammatory medications are an essential part of the therapy approach. Again, benzoyl peroxide is a good and low-cost alternative in this situation. Scrubbing, dermabrasion, and power washing brushes, among other things, might cause increased inflammation and should be avoided.

Disordered desquamation or sloughing is frequently the least understood cause of acne. When your skin renews itself, new cells are generated in the dermis and develop slowly from the skin's bottom layer to the epidermis. The adult epidermal cells are eventually sloughed off and replaced from below. When the time comes for those skin cells to be sloughed off, the connections between the cells may not break readily, causing the cells to come off irregularly or too slowly, resulting in pore blockage, thickening of the top layer, and other problems. This causes oil gland obstruction, oil backup, bacterial proliferation, irritation, infection, and severe outbreaks. The goal is to keep the epidermis sloughing off in a regular and even manner. Retinols and acids can be used to treat desquamation disorders (alpha and beta hydroxy acids, salicylic acid, lactic acid, etc.). Chemical peels can speed up the sloughing process, while topical retinol or acids can keep it going. Retinols may be extremely irritating if taken at high concentrations; therefore, I recommend low dosage, delayed-release retinol at night, with the amount gradually increasing over time if tolerated. Accutane is the grandfather of all retinoids because it both dries up oil and produces considerable continuing sloughing, which is why it is so successful in treating acne. Wherever feasible, acne management strategies should include parts of therapy that target all four causes.

Once acne is under control and outbreaks are fewer and less severe, the long-term detrimental consequences of acne can be addressed. This includes the common redness, hyperpigmentation, and scarring associated with severe acne.

IPL is frequently used to address redness and hyperpigmentation (intense pulse light therapy). Typically, three or four treatments are required. Chemical peels can also be beneficial in this regard. Mild to moderate scarring may frequently be healed with micro-needling treatments, but more significant scars (depressed or ice pick scars) are best addressed with fractionated lasers such as Fraxel Dual, which can help improve hyperpigmentation.

What is acne?

Our visible pores connect to oil glands (officially known as sebaceous glands) beneath the skin through hair follicles, which discharge sebum to the skin's surface to maintain its supple and avoid dryness.

When there is an excess of sebum generated, it can clog and plug the follicles with dead skin and debris, resulting in the appearance of familiar friends: blackheads and whiteheads. When pores get clogged, they can become inflamed or infected, resulting in furious pimples in the form of papules and pustules or, in extreme cases, nodules and cysts. Acne does not just affect the face; it may also affect other parts of the body, such as the back and chest.

Acne vulgaris is a common skin condition caused by an accumulation of oils, skin cells, and other debris in the hair follicle. Acne is caused by inflammation and the proliferation of certain kinds of bacteria.

Acne is more prevalent in adolescents and young adults, but it may afflict people of all ages. Frequently afflicted areas include the face, neck, chest, upper back, and upper arms.

Mild acne is distinguished by noninflamed lesions with no or few inflamed pimples, whereas severe acne is distinguished by inflamed cysts and nodules.

1

What Causes Acne?

Acne is essentially a hormonal disease caused by male or 'androgenic' hormones that become active throughout the adolescent years. Acne is caused by sensitivity to such hormones, in conjunction with germs on the skin and fatty acids within oil glands. Acne is more common on the face, chest, shoulders, neck, and back, where oil glands are located.

Acne is caused primarily by increased sebum production, hormonal factors, bacterial colonization, and inflammation. Sebum is an oily substance generated by sebaceous glands situated surrounding hair follicles. Excessive sebum production gives bacteria a nutrient-rich environment in which to thrive. Cutibacterium acnes (C. acnes; previously P. acnes) is the bacteria that cause inflammatory acne when it collects in a pore.

The presence of germs alone can activate the immune system, resulting in inflammation. Inflammation aggravates acne and further destroys the skin.

Hormones have a role as well. Androgens are hormones that are released by the testicles, ovaries, adrenal glands, and fat cells. Changes in these hormones can increase sebum production and lead to acne development. Acne can be exacerbated by androgen excess conditions such as polycystic ovarian syndrome (a large number of abnormal cysts in the ovaries).

Risk Factors

Acne development and severity can be influenced by a number of risk factors. These variables do not cause acne on their own, but they might aggravate it.

Genetics: According to studies, people with first-degree family members who have acne are more than three times more likely to develop it than people who do not have afflicted family members. This implies that genetics have a significant influence on the development of acne.

Diet: Acne worsening has been associated with high glycemic load diets (poor nutritional value and excessive carbohydrates such as sweetened drinks, white rice, and french fries).

Although many individuals assume that chocolate causes acne, no conclusive evidence has been found.

Smoking: Smokers are more prone to acquire acne and to suffer from severe acne. There is also a dose-dependent link, which indicates that the more cigarettes a person smokes, the more likely they are to develop or aggravate acne.

Stress: Acne severity can be exacerbated by emotional stress.

Whiteheads, blackheads, tiny bumps, nodules, and cysts are all examples of acne lesions.

Though acne is a natural physiologic occurrence, some circumstances can worsen it, including:
- Hormone levels fluctuate around the time of menstruation (women).
- Acne lesions are being manipulated (picked/prodded).
- Clothing and headgear (for example, hats and sports helmets).

Causes of Adult Acne

You're probably over the difficulties that caused your adolescent acne by now, right? Your random breakouts, on the other hand, may imply differently.

Acne is frequently caused by puberty. It affects around 8 out of every 10 preteens and teenagers. But hormones aren't the sole cause of those bothersome pimples. So, if you thought your first crush left you with breakouts and pimples, think again.

According to the American Academy of Dermatology, up to 15% of adult women experience acne (AAD). "What's intriguing is that you may develop it [as an adult] even if you didn't have it when you were a teenager," explains Francesca Fusco, MD, an assistant clinical professor of dermatology at Mount Sinai Medical Center in New York City.

Although the pimples appear to be the same, adult breakouts differ from those seen in high school. "Adult acne is often seen on the bottom part of the face, whereas teen acne is frequently found on the top half," Dr. Fusco explains. "Adult acne is also deeper and manifests itself as cysts or 'under the skin' pimples that cannot be drained." Cosmetics, your skin-care routine, and lifestyle choices, as well as variables you've never considered, might all be to fault.

Learn about the surprising reasons for your adult acne, whether it's due to hairspray or travel.

1. Hairstyling products that come into contact with your skin might aggravate acne.

Breakouts induced by hair-care products are so prevalent that they've earned their own moniker: pomade acne. "Styling creams ooze oil onto the forehead, trapping acne-causing bacteria in your pores," explains Richard Fried, MD, Ph.D., director of Yardley

Dermatology Associates in Yardley, Pennsylvania, and author of the book Healing Adult Acne.

When pores get clogged, they become irritated, resulting in redness, pus, and, eventually, blackheads and whiteheads along the hairline and forehead.

Your hairdo is also important: Bangs aggravate acne by pushing skin-clogging hair products right up against your brow.
"What you use on your hair often ends up on your face, especially if you use spray applicators," Dr. Fried adds.

Use your hands to apply cosmetics and keep them away from your hairline. After applying, use a face cleanser to remove any excess styling product from your skin.

2. In an unexpected way, facial hair removal can lead to acne.

You're exchanging one complexion issue — facial hair — for another: rough skin.

According to Fusco, topical treatments applied to your skin before or after hair removal might be comedogenic (meaning they block pores and encourage acne). Itchy bumps following hair removal may not be real acne, but rather "an inflammation of the hair follicle that creates a temporary rash," she adds.

Apply a warm compress to your face three to four times each day to relieve the rash. Consult your doctor if this does not work. To get rid of the rash, you may need to take an antibiotic. Clean hairy areas before de-fuzzing to decrease germs on your skin, and use non-comedogenic products that will not clog your pores.

3. Using too many skin-care products can exacerbate acne.

Every year, you might try out a few new skin-care products. That's great for the cosmetics business, but it's terrible for your skin.

Switching or adding a new product before giving it a chance to work "challenges your skin with new preservatives and active ingredients, which can be irritating and cause breakouts," according to Paul Jarrod Frank, MD, the founder and director of Fifth Avenue Dermatology Surgery and Laser Center in New York.

And here's a surprise: Even anti-acne products might create pimples if used excessively. "I have acne patients who use four or five different acne creams or an astringent, face wash, and spot cream, all with acne-fighting ingredients," Dr. Frank adds. "It rips their flesh apart."

Whether you want to combat wrinkles or get rid of zits, choose one or two products and let them four to six weeks to work. "It takes that long for the skin to flip over," Frank adds. Do you need another reason to avoid experimenting with acne "cures"? You'll save money at the pharmacy and have more room in your medication cabinet.

4. Acne may be exacerbated by your makeup remover (or lack thereof).

Cosmetics that clog your pores might mix with your natural skin oil to create acne cosmetic outbreaks. Frank says that the issue isn't just with the items but also with how they're removed.

"Either ladies clean their skin in a perfunctory manner, or they believe they don't need to wash their face fully since they're using mineral makeup," he says.

Makeup, grease, and grime accumulate after a long day. This is a three-pronged attack that may easily block your pores, trapping acne-causing germs and creating outbreaks.

Choose non-comedogenic products and wash your face thoroughly — and gently — every night. Apply makeup gently, clean your makeup brushes once a week, and don't share cosmetic items.

5. Traveling to a new location may wreak havoc on your skin and contribute to breakouts.

Have you ever wondered why your skin appears like the moon's surface after a vacation? Acne can be triggered by changes in the environment, such as the sun, heat, and humidity.

"Your skin isn't used to such substances, so it is challenged and reacts by breaking out," Frank explains. Zit remover You can't control the temperature or humidity where you go, but avoiding excessive sun exposure and applying sunscreen with zinc oxide or titanium dioxide may help minimize outbreaks. And, because your skin is adjusting to environmental changes, don't add to the epidermal stress by introducing new products.

6. Sunscreens with higher SPF levels may promote acne breakouts.

If you have acne-prone skin, you should always use sunscreen, but which sunscreen is best for you? "People with acne or acne-prone skin should search for oil-free, non-comedogenic sunscreens," advises Yoram Harth, MD, medical director of MDacne in San Francisco. He claims that "heavier" sunscreens that aren't labeled as oil-free might clog skin pores and create more acne.

There are two types of active chemicals in sunscreens. Chemical compounds that soak into the skin and protect against damaging UV radiation, as well as physical agents (also known as mineral sunscreens) that sit on the skin's surface to form a sun shield.

Because they deflect the sun's rays, physical sunscreens are frequently advised for sensitive skin. These sunscreens, however, can be thicker, leaving a white cast on the face and potentially blocking pores, whereas chemical sunscreens are undetectable, very light, and leave the skin shine-free, according to Dr. Harth.

If you get acne after applying physical sunscreen, you may need to use a thinner product. Change to a sunscreen that contains chemical compounds such as avobenzone, oxybenzone, methoxycinnamate, or octocrylene. Also, after a day in the sun, remember to wash your sunscreen off your skin. Even the lightest, most transparent sunscreens can block pores if left on overnight.

7. Acne may be caused by a diet high in processed foods and refined carbohydrates.

As teenagers, we thought fatty food and chocolate cake were to blame for our acne. That may still be true for you now that you're an adult.

According to Fusco, "the most recent scientific research shows that high-carbohydrate diets may predispose you to acne." More study is needed; however, diets heavy in refined carbohydrates ("white" foods such as white bread and white pasta, as well as crackers, cake, and cookies) that are high on the glycemic index may enhance the onset and severity of breakouts. The glycemic index is a scale that measures how much a particular diet affects blood sugar levels.

According to Harth, there may possibly be a relationship between acne and dairy.

According to Harth, "dairy products have been proven in several studies to raise levels of insulin-like growth factor, which can cause or exacerbate acne breakouts." Cow's milk, especially low-fat milk, which has a high quantity of progesterone-like hormones and has a greater sugar content than full-fat milk, is one of the most triggering kinds of dairy. Reduce your intake of snacks such as chips and ice cream in favor of whole grains, vegetables, fruits, and high-protein meals.

8. Stress causes hormonal changes that increase your risk of acne.

Are you worried about a big project's approaching deadline? Do you have problems in your relationship that keep you up at night? Stress does not cause breakouts, but it may make them worse.

"Stress can aggravate acne by causing the production of inflammatory substances known as neuropeptides and hormonal changes," Fried explains. Even "positive" stress, like preparing for a major event, can cause breakouts. This is why a large pimple appears on your wedding day or before a major date.

To clean up stress-related outbreaks, use acne treatments containing salicylic acid and benzoyl peroxide. Find a technique to soothe your anxieties, whether it's yoga, deep breathing, or watching a chick film, to avoid future flareups.

9. Cell phones have the potential to spread acne-causing bacteria to your face.

All of that on-the-go talking is fantastic for staying in contact with friends, family, and coworkers. But what about your skin tone? Not at all.

"Throughout the day, you expose your mobile phone to bacteria-infested surfaces, and when you chat on the phone, you bring this bacteria near to your lips," Fusco explains.

Furthermore, touching your mobile phone (or conventional phone, for that matter) against your face might create "acne mechanica," which is pimples caused by friction. Bacteria can also be transferred when you touch your face after texting on your phone.

Allow your phone to rest every now and again, and clean it with an alcohol wipe on a regular basis.

10. Dry skin, like oily skin, is a potential cause of acne breakouts.

True, oily skin is a source of severe breakouts, but so is the opposite extreme. Fusco explains that "dry skin might have tiny cracks and fissures in which bacteria can proliferate and produce acne." Furthermore, dry skin flakes can block pores.

Exfoliate your skin gently a few times each week, then hydrate with a non-comedogenic moisturizer designed for dry skin.

2

Types of Acne

The two major kinds of acne vulgaris, inflammatory and non-inflammatory, reflect the disease's range. The most severe type of acne is inflammatory acne.

Non-Inflammatory acne

Non-inflammatory acne, also known as comedonal acne, develops when sebum and dead skin cells build up in the pilosebaceous unit (the hair follicles and associated oil glands). Comedones can be closed (whiteheads) or open (blackheads) (blackheads).

Microcomedones

Microcomedones (tiny blocked pores) develop when sebum and keratin begin to clog skin pores. Microcomedones are the first acne lesions and are usually not noticeable.

Closed comedones or whiteheads

Closed comedones or whiteheads form as microcomedones grow. They have white cores and maybe hair growing from them. Whiteheads should not be popped because they do not contain pus or fluid.

Open comedones or blackheads

A whitehead can open up with continuing enlargement, revealing the substance inside and transforming it into a blackhead or open comedones. The black hue of open comedones are caused by the oxidation of cellular waste and lipids, as well as the accumulation of dead cells and the pigment melanin.

Inflammatory acne

Acne is caused by bacterial colonization, which can encourage the immune system to produce an inflammatory response. The severity of inflammatory acne lesions is related to the degree of inflammation.

Papules

Papules are the first inflammatory lesions that appear when a comedo becomes inflamed. They are elevated, sensitive, tiny bumps that range in hue from pink to red.

Pustules

Pustules are big, painful skin lumps that contain pus. Because of the pus, the core of a pustule is white or yellowish, and it may be surrounded by swelling and redness.

Pimples

Pimples are not a distinct form of acne lesion–the term "pimple" refers to any tiny inflammatory lesion. Pimples are commonly used to describe papules and pustules.

Nodules

A nodule develops when germs, debris, and inflammatory cells seep into the surrounding skin from a damaged follicle. Nodules are painful, deep-seated lumps that are extremely inflamed and difficult to touch.

Cysts

Cysts are highly inflammatory lesions that contain a lot of pus. They are unpleasant and delicate to the touch and can be white or red in color. When cysts appear alongside nodules, the condition is known as nodulocystic acne. Because nodulocystic and cystic acne is the most severe kinds of acne, they are the most prone to cause skin scarring.

3

The Signs and Symptoms of Acne

Acne symptoms begin with a clogged pore, which leads to a lesion on the skin. This might include everything from non-inflamed bumps and blackheads to inflamed, red pimples and pustules. Cystic acne has the most severe symptoms, which can result in scarring.

Frequent Symptoms

Acne's main symptom is blemished, which you may plainly see or feel on yourself, your children, or other individuals in your care. Most people have blemishes that are both non-inflamed and inflamed. Acne blemishes are most commonly seen on the face, although acne can also form on the neck, chest, shoulders, back, and buttocks.

Non-Inflamed Acne Symptoms

Non-inflamed acne, also known as comedonal acne, does not produce red or painful blemishes. Non-inflamed acne symptoms include lumps or bumpiness over the skin's surface, as well as uneven skin texture. The lesions are comedones, which are clogged skin pores that can be open (blackheads) or closed (whiteheads) (milia or whiteheads). Even though comedones are not visible, they will cause the skin to feel rough or sandpaper-like.

Acne outbreaks that are not inflammatory include:
- Pimples and blackheads (open comedones).
- Milia (non-inflamed whiteheads).
- Comedones that are closed (non-inflamed bumps).
- Microcomedones (pore blockages too small to see).

Inflamed Acne Symptoms

Acne breakouts that are inflamed result in red, puffy pimples. Inflamed acne might be minor, with only a few breakouts here and there, or it can be severe, with deep lesions. These blemishes can leak, crust, and scab over in addition to being bloated.

Common symptoms of inflamed acne outbreaks include:
- Papules are tiny lumps on the skin (red, raised bumps that may be small or large).
- Pustules are a kind of pustule that appears on the skin (red, inflamed, with a white head).

While nodules and cysts are less frequent kinds of inflammatory acne lesions, they can be found in more severe cases. Nodules and cysts are bigger than a regular pimple and grow in deeper layers of the skin.

Timing of Breakouts

Acne outbreaks are frequently associated with hormonal levels, which is why they occur throughout the adolescent years. Acne outbreaks are frequent in women in the week preceding menstruation and can last till menopause. Acne breakouts are common in pregnant women.

Rare Symptoms

The most severe kind of inflammatory acne is cystic acne. Acne cysts and nodules that are considerable in quantity and severity develop in people with nodulocystic acne.

- Acne cysts have the appearance of soft, fluid-filled, uncomfortable lumps beneath the skin's surface.
- Acne nodules are hard, painful bumps beneath the skin's surface. It takes a long time for them to heal.

Complications/Sub-Group Indications

Acne can cause problems and may be of particular concern in some groups.

Excoriated Acne

Picking at or scratching your acne lesions (or imagined lesions) to the extent of injuring the skin causes excoriated acne. This issue is more common in women, and it may be related to obsessive/compulsive excoriation disease.

Squeezing or picking at the skin all the time results in angry red pimples, open red sores, scratches, crusts, and scabs. This can develop into a nodule or cyst.

Post-Inflammatory Hyperpigmentation

The medical name for dark, discolored patches that remain after an acne blemish has healed is post-inflammatory hyperpigmentation. It's a fairly common condition, and most acne sufferers will get these markings to some extent. Fortunately, post-inflammatory hyperpigmentation is not a real scar and will usually disappear with time.

Scarring

Inflamed acne outbreaks frequently result in depressed or pitted scarring, sometimes known as ice pick scars (long, narrow impressions in the skin). Acne blemishes can also create hypertrophic, or raised, scars in certain persons.

Acne in People With Diabetes

People with diabetes are more likely to experience inflamed acne outbreaks because they have a lower tolerance to skin and soft tissue infections. Some prescription acne medications, such as Zenatane (isotretinoin, a vitamin A derivative), may have an effect on blood sugar levels, and your doctor may want to constantly monitor you if you use these.

Acne in Pregnant Women

A woman may acquire acne or have a fresh breakout as a result of the hormonal changes during pregnancy. Some prescription acne medications are not advised to be used during pregnancy since they might cross the placenta and cause birth abnormalities, miscarriage, and stillbirth.4

4

Acne Myths

Cleanse, Cleanse, Cleanse

Acne is not always caused by poor hygiene, and over-cleansing can irritate sensitive areas worse than, so be cautious and choose essential treatments to target. Exfoliants, because of their abrasive nature, may induce further irritation. To avoid spreading dirt or bacteria, wash your hands before and after your skincare regimen, and avoid touching your face excessively during the day.

Squeeze, Squeeze, Squeeze

Squeezing pimples, especially those that are firmly embedded beneath the skin, can result in scarring, which needs additional therapy and attention. It can also promote the spread of acne-causing germs, therefore REFUSE THE URGE. Ingredients like Succinic Acid and Salicylic Acid can help unclog pores and decrease oil, which can aid in the treatment of acne and outbreaks.

Only teenagers get acne

Acne makes no distinctions based on age, gender, or color. It may be more prevalent among teens owing to hormonal changes, but it is by no means exclusive. Sebum imbalance can be caused by changes in food, environment, and hormone fluctuations during pregnancy/menstruation.

Toothpaste can cure your acne

It's a tried-and-true DIY tip passed down through generations, but the fluoride in toothpaste can be harmful to the skin. Salicylic acid, for example, has been shown to be more helpful in clearing blemishes, so reserve the paste for those pearly whites.

Chocolate causes acne

Finally, some good news: there is little to no scientific evidence that chocolate has a direct influence on acne outbreaks or severity. That is not to rule out diet in general, since there is a chance that specific food categories may affect an individual's acne symptoms. Therefore it is always worth discussing with a doctor or dermatologist.

Acne normally happens to people with oily skin

Acne and breakouts, as we've seen, come in a variety of ways. Sure, oily skin produces more extra oil, which is a crucial component in the breakout recipe, but it is not the only one. Knowing your skin type is a fantastic method to avoid breakouts by integrating items to maintain it in balance, such as regulating oil production and moisturizing dry areas, into your daily regimen.

5

Treatments

Acne Treatments

Acne treatment methods include topical creams, oral medicines, and specialized medical gadgets. To maximize acne therapy, the American Academy of Dermatology suggests mixing more than one treatment component.

Over the counter topicals

Benzoyl peroxide, salicylic acid, alpha-hydroxy acids, and sulfur are examples of topical acne treatments available without a prescription.

Benzoyl peroxide is a topical medicine that has antibacterial characteristics as well as the capacity to dissolve comedones. It has the ability to remove excess sebum and dead skin cells. Because salicylic acid is a lipid-soluble substance, it can get deep into the follicles. It can unclog pores and alleviate comedones by slowing down the shedding of dead skin cells.

Alpha-hydroxy acids, such as glycolic acid, are popular skin anti-aging treatments. Glycolic and lactic acids can help acne by decreasing dead skin cell shedding and combating skin color changes caused by inflammation.

Although sulfur has been used to treat acne for many years, the data supporting its efficacy is limited. It is frequently used in conjunction with other medicines such as benzoyl peroxide and sulfacetamide. Sulfur is considered to function by eliminating dead skin cells and limiting C. acnes bacterial reproduction.

Prescription topicals

Topical retinoids, topical antibiotics, and azelaic acid are examples of topical acne treatments that require a doctor's prescription to purchase.

Retinoids, such as isotretinoin, are vitamin A derivatives that help reduce skin cell shedding, clear pores, prevent the development of microcomedones, and reduce inflammation. In the United States, prescription topical retinoids include tretinoin (0.02-0.08 percent), tazarotene (0.05-0.1 percent), and adapalene (0.3 percent). Differin (adapalene 0.1 percent gel) is available without a prescription.

C. acnes, the acne-causing bacterium, can be killed or inhibited by antibiotics. Azelaic acid contains comedolytic (comedone-breaking) effects, as well as antibacterial and anti-inflammatory qualities. Azelaic acid is available in 15% and 20% concentrations; however only the 20% version is FDA-approved for acne therapy.

Oral isotretinoin

Oral isotretinoin is a prescription-only retinoid used to treat severe acne or acne that has become resistant to therapy. It reduces inflammation by lowering sebum production, suppressing C. acnes, and inhibiting sebum production.

In individuals with severe acne, three to four months of isotretinoin treatment can result in a 60-95 percent decrease in inflammatory lesions. Isotretinoin capsules containing 8 to 40 mg of isotretinoin are available for oral use.

Antibiotics

Antibiotics are an essential part of acne treatment regimens. Antibiotics combat the bacterial component of acne, and some have anti-inflammatory effects. Acne can be effectively treated with both topical and oral antibiotics.

Antibiotics are applied to acne lesions or taken orally once or twice daily. They are generally given for three to four months, following which your dermatologist will determine whether or not you should continue taking them.

Clindamycin, erythromycin, dapsone, minocycline, and sulfacetamide are examples of topical acne antibiotics. Tetracyclines (e.g., doxycycline), macrolides (e.g., erythromycin and azithromycin), trimethoprim-sulfamethoxazole, and amoxicillin are examples of oral antibiotics.

Professional treatments

Professional acne treatments in the office include photodynamic therapy, chemical peels, microdermabrasion, and comedone extraction.

Photodynamic treatment includes applying a photosensitive substance to the skin, such as aminolevulinic acid (ALA), and then subjecting it to a laser or other specific light source. Theoretically, photodynamic treatment reduces sebum production by inhibiting C. acnes and injuring sebaceous glands.

In those with non-inflamed comedonal acne, superficial chemical peels may hasten comedo resolution. Peeling chemicals that are most often utilized include glycolic acid and salicylic acid. Microdermabrasion is a non-invasive treatment that exfoliates the skin with microscopic needles. The mechanical removal of comedones by a tiny incision under a local anesthetic is known as comedo extraction.

DIY at-home treatments

Although there is some evidence that at-home therapies can help with acne, there is not enough data to recommend their usage instead of standard acne treatments.

Topical tea tree oil was proven to be helpful in treating mild-to-moderate acne in one research. Another research compared topical tea tree oil to benzoyl peroxide and found that both treatments improved skin, although tea tree oil was slower to generate results. People suffering from mild-to-moderate acne may benefit from using green tea lotion to their skin. After six weeks of twice-daily usage of green tea lotion, one research found a 58 percent reduction in the number of lesions.

Medication

If self-care does not assist your acne, there are a few over-the-counter acne medicines available. The majority of these medicines have chemicals that can aid in the killing of germs or the reduction of oil on your skin. These are some examples:

Many acne treatments and gels include benzoyl peroxide. It's utilized to get rid of existing pimples and prevent the formation of new ones. Benzoyl peroxide also kills acne-causing microorganisms. Sulfur is a natural ingredient that has a distinct odor and may be found in a number of lotions, cleansers, and masks. Resorcinol is a chemical that is less frequently employed in the elimination of dead skin cells.

Salicylic acid may be found in a variety of soaps and acne treatments. It helps to keep pores from becoming blocked. You may continue to have symptoms at times. If this occurs, you should seek medical attention. Your doctor may be able to give medicines to assist in alleviating your discomfort and avoid scarring. These are some examples:

Antibiotics, whether taken orally or used topically, decrease inflammation and kill the germs that cause pimples. Antibiotics are typically only taken for a limited period of time to prevent your body from developing resistance and leaving you susceptible to infections.

Prescription topical creams, such as retinoic acid or prescription-strength benzoyl peroxide, are frequently more effective than over-the-counter therapies. They are working to minimize the amount of oil produced. Benzoyl peroxide is a bactericidal agent that inhibits acne-causing bacteria from developing antibiotic resistance. It also possesses mild comedones-dissolving and anti-inflammatory effects. Birth control tablets or spironolactone may be used to treat hormonal acne in women. These medicines control hormones that cause acne by reducing oil production.

Isotretinoin (Accutane) is a vitamin-A-based medicine that is used to treat severe nodular acne. It has significant adverse effects and is only used after other therapies have failed. Your doctor may advise you on treatments to treat severe acne and avoid scarring. These treatments function by eliminating damaged skin and decreasing oil production.

They are as follows:

Photodynamic therapy: To decrease oil production and microorganisms, medicine and a specific light or laser are used. Other lasers can be used on their own to aid with acne or scars.

Dermabrasion: removes the top layers of your skin with a spinning brush and is ideal for reducing acne scars rather than treating acne itself.

Microdermabrasion: is a gentler treatment that aids in the removal of dead skin cells.

The top layers of your skin are removed using a chemical peel. That skin peels away, revealing less damaged skin beneath. Mild acne scars can be improved with chemical peels.

If your acne is characterized by big cysts, your doctor may advise you to use cortisone injections. Cortisol is a steroid that your body naturally produces. It has the ability to decrease inflammation and accelerate recovery. Cortisone is typically used in conjunction with other acne treatments.

Tips to manage acne

In addition to taking acne treatments that have been shown to be beneficial, such as retinoids and antibiotics, you can improve your acne by adopting certain lifestyle modifications. Proper skincare, nutritional modifications, and stress reduction are all significant variables that can aid with healing and breakout management.

Proper skincare

Acne patients' skincare is aimed at preventing irritation. Following these guidelines will help you maintain your skin's health and cleanliness without causing damage to it:
Instead of soap, use a synthetic detergent cleaner (syndet) like Cetaphil. Syndet cleansers have a pH range of 5.5 to 7, which is closer to the pH of normal skin than ordinary soap.

Avoid cleaning your skin too hard or picking at your acne blemishes. Mechanical damage caused by vigorous treatment of the lesions can induce inflammation and scarring. Oil-free, water-based cosmetics are non-comedogenic, so use these instead of oil-based products. Wash your face with warm–not hot–water on a frequent basis, especially after sweating. Excessive sun exposure and tanning beds can harm your skin and cause irritation. Some acne medicines might make your skin more sunburned.

Diet modification

Several studies have found that high glycemic load diets and excessive milk intake may lead to acne.

Although more study is needed to establish the link between acne and food, many experts advocate transitioning to a healthy low glycemic load diet and limiting milk and dairy consumption.

Stress reduction

Acne severity has been connected to psychological stress. Stress-reduction techniques such as meditation and regular exercise may help your acne.

Acne Scarring

Scarring occurs as a result of abnormal wound healing, which is more likely to exacerbate inflammatory acne lesions. Acne scars can be atrophic (tissue loss that shows as indentations) or hypertrophic (tissue growth) (excess collagen resulting in elevated scars). Scarring affects around 1% of acne patients. Laser resurfacing, chemical peels, dermabrasion, injectable soft tissue fillers, steroid injections, cryotherapy (freezing), and surgical excision are among treatment options for acne scars.Acne is a common skin disorder characterized by the appearance of multiple lesions on the face, neck, and upper torso. It is caused by a combination of follicle clogging with oil, bacterial overgrowth, and inflammation, and is exacerbated by stress, smoking, and poor nutrition.

With therapy, most people may completely recover from acne. Prescription and over-the-counter medicines, antibiotics, and professional treatments like as laser resurfacing and chemical peels are all available as therapy alternatives. Changes in lifestyle can assist to reduce the severity of acne.

6

Finding Adult Treatment for Acne

You've probably tried every lotion, elixir, and serum on the market in search of an efficient adult acne cure. However, it also aids in getting to the source of the problem. To put it another way, in order to truly cure adult acne, you may need to first understand what causes it in the first place.

Because there's nothing more depressing than waiting until your 20s to finally have clear skin, only to discover the hard way that severe breakouts don't necessarily stop when your adolescent years do. Coming to grips with adult acne is difficult—but don't worry, you're not the only one.

What causes breakouts?

A clogged pore is at the core of all acne. Because they contain your sebaceous glands, your pores, which are the openings that surround each hair follicle, are an important component of your skin.

Through the pore opening, these glands produce sebum (oil), which helps keep your skin smooth and protected. However, clogging the pore with debris, dead skin cells, excess oil, and perhaps germs is a formula for a pimple.

Simply taking better care of your skin by cleansing and exfoliating on a regular basis might sometimes be enough to keep acne at bay. However, for many others, the situation is more difficult. And, especially if you're an adult, figuring out what's causing your acne may be quite difficult.

Best adult acne treatment strategies

1. Topical treatments with acne-fighting ingredients

The first and most crucial step in treating acne is to stock your medicine cabinet with medicines containing scientifically proven components. Remember that not every product or ingredient will work for everyone, and many of these items will require you to use them consistently for a few weeks before you notice any difference in your skin. So go slowly—but persistently if you're not experiencing any improvements or can't locate items that don't bother your skin, consult a dermatologist for advice and, perhaps, a prescription therapy.

The following are the components to search for:

Salicylic acid is a kind of chemical exfoliator known as a beta-hydroxy acid (BHA). It works by breaking the connections that hold dead skin cells together. Salicylic acid is also particularly beneficial in the treatment of acne since it is oil-soluble, allowing it to work its unclogging magic deeper into your greasy pores than other chemical exfoliants.

It may be found in a variety of over-the-counter cleansers, spot treatments, and masks. It's mild enough to apply on your entire face—possibly even daily—for the majority of individuals. To begin, use a cleanser containing salicylic acid.

Glycolic acid is another form of chemical exfoliator that is an alpha-hydroxy acid (AHA).

It can be found in cleansers, serums, and peels. Pay attention to the amount of glycolic acid in a product since this will tell you how potent it is. As the concentration increases, the substance becomes more potent but also more sensitizing.

Lactic acid is another type of chemical exfoliator known as an AHA. However, lactic acid is regarded to be milder than other forms of chemical exfoliants, so if you're new to exfoliating treatments, it's an excellent place to start.

Found in: Lactic acid is frequently combined with other acids in serums, toners, and peels, which means you might be exposed to a stronger acid without realizing it.

Another kind of chemical exfoliant is polyhydroxy acids (PHAs), which include gluconolactone and lactobionic acid. PHAs are usually thought to be the gentlest. If you have really dry or sensitive skin, or if you've had negative responses to other chemical exfoliants in the past, you should think about using a PHA.

It may be found in a variety of exfoliating peels, masks, and lotions.

Benzoyl peroxide helps by eliminating the acne bacteria while also exfoliating the pores. It is not as mild as chemical exfoliants, so use caution and hydrate afterward.

Found in: PanOxyl face cleanser is a traditional derm suggestion that comes in both lower and higher strength variants. However, benzoyl peroxide is also available in numerous lotions and spot treatments, where it is frequently combined with a chemical exfoliator like salicylic acid.

Sulfur may not have as much evidence behind it for acne as some of the other choices on our list, but it is frequently suggested as a therapy for rosacea-related acne-like blemishes.

Found in: Spot treatments and face masks are the most common.

Azelaic acid is another rosacea/acne crossover drug that is effective at removing rosacea bumps as well as pimples. As previously stated by SELF, the specific mechanism by which azelaic acid acts is not completely understood. We do know, however, that it is effective.

Found in: Azelaic acid is accessible in a few prescription forms, although it is also found in lesser amounts in over-the-counter treatments.

Retinoids, which include retinol, retinal (retinaldehyde), and retinoic acid, are vitamin A derivatives. They are available as over-the-counter (retinol is generally the active component in these) and stronger prescription forms. "Topical retinoids are luckily one of the most efficient acne treatments, as well as a highly effective anti-aging ingredient," Dr. Tzu says.

The main disadvantage is that they are abrasive and can sometimes be too much for delicate skin, especially when you first start using them. That is why, at first, it is critical to use them only a few times each week, to constantly moisturize well, and to be particularly vigilant about wearing sunscreen when taking a retinoid.

Found in: Retinol is available in a variety of over-the-counter medications, which is usually the best place to start because retinoids may be unpleasant.

2. Exfoliators

"The most essential thing you can do on a regular basis to battle acne, both in terms of prevention and treatment," Dr. Schultz adds. Whether you use a chemical or manual exfoliator, this step will help prevent breakouts by keeping your pores free and removing any blockages you may have.

Dr. Schultz recommends glycolic acid as a go-to component if your skin can tolerate it, and he recommends utilizing leave-on treatments like masks rather than cleansers, which only stay on your skin for a limited period of time.

However, be cautious not to exfoliate too frequently since this might result in irritated, flaky, dry skin. Most individuals can tolerate one to three times per week. However, your skin may be able to tolerate more or less depending on your specific skin type and problems.

3. Spot treatments

Spot treatments, particularly those containing benzoyl peroxide, are essential for treating a pimple as soon as possible since they operate by eliminating the bacteria that is frequently responsible for acne. It might be a touch abrasive, so people with sensitive skin should use caution.

4. Products that fight inflammation

As previously stated, pimples occur when a pore becomes clogged with debris, oil, or dead skin cells. If germs are present, the pimple may become inflamed, turning red, puffy, and painful. Not all pimples are inflamed, but those that are especially painful to deal with. So it's critical to discover strategies to calm them down while also addressing the core cause of the problem.

If you have inflamed acne, seek products that have soothing ingredients (such as colloidal oatmeal, aloe, or Centella Asiatica) as well as acne-fighting chemicals such as salicylic acid.

5. Oral medications

Depending on the underlying cause(s) and severity of your acne, you may discover that topical therapies are ineffective. For example, hormonal acne is caused by internal processes that cannot be controlled by external medicines.

In that situation, your dermatologist may advise you to take oral medicine. "Medications that regulate hormone levels, such as oral contraceptives and spironolactone, can help reduce hormonal chin and lower face outbreaks," adds Dr. Tzu. Furthermore, oral retinoids such as isotretinoin (previously Accutane) are regarded as the main dermatological weapons in the fight against acne.

Inquire with your dermatologist about what could work best for you.

6. Cortisone injections

Topical therapies are unlikely to be effective in the treatment of cystic acne. And because those large, painful zits are so deep in the skin, picking and prodding at them is more likely to leave a scar than other types of acne. "The only way to reduce it quickly is to drain it, which is not a do-it-yourself project," Dr. Schultz warns.

If you have access to a dermatologist, one option for dealing with a persistent cyst is to have a cortisone shot. "Cortisone injections are real 'spot treatments' for severe cystic acne lesions," explains Dr. Tzu.

However, you can treat them at home by applying a warm or cold compress (whichever feels better to you), a small amount of over-the-counter hydrocortisone cream to reduce inflammation, and simply waiting it out.

Other highly effective adult acne treatments and habits for clear and glowing skin

Pimples, no matter how old you are, generally form in the same time-honored way: Pores, which contain oil glands, get clogged, allowing dirt, germs, and cells to accumulate and create a blockage.

Hormonal changes, either during the monthly cycle or during a menopausal transition, are the most common cause for most women. Adult acne flare-ups are also caused by nutritional imbalances and stress.

Reduce your intake of processed carbohydrates.

According to dermatologist Albert Lefkovits, MD, of the Park Avenue Center for Advanced Medical and Cosmetic Dermatology in

New York City, "eating chocolate or a lot of junk food does not seem to cause acne by itself."

According to a 2016 review of studies on how food impacts acne, "compelling evidence indicates that high glycemic load diets may exacerbate acne," according to the researchers. More refined carbs, such as white bread, have a high glycemic index (GI). Scientists believe that carbohydrate-induced insulin increases may cause the release of hormones that inflame follicles and boost oil production.

In one 2018 study, researchers randomly assigned 66 individuals to a high GI or lower GI diet for two weeks. They discovered that those who ate low GI meals had lower levels of IGF-1, a hormone that is known to cause acne outbreaks.

If you suspect your diet is to blame, avoid the following high GI foods (those with a GI of 70 or higher) and see if you notice a difference: sugary snacks and beverages, white bread, bagels, corn flakes, instant oatmeal, white rice, potatoes, pretzels, popcorn, and certain fruits, such as watermelon.

Consume less diary

While more study is needed to fully understand how dairy consumption may contribute to acne, a growing body of evidence shows a relationship, according to the American Academy of Dermatology.

According to a 2018 meta-analysis published in the Journal of the European Academy of Dermatology and Venereology, milk consumption—particularly skim milk, which is richer in sugar than whole milk—was related to an increased incidence of acne. Aside from the increased sugar level, experts believe that proteins and hormones contained in milk products, such as IGF-1, may contribute to acne flare-ups by boosting oil production and inflammation.

Surprisingly, yogurt and cheese do not appear to have the same impact, according to a 2018 meta-analysis published in the journal Clinical Nutrition.

So, if you consume milk on a daily basis, try switching to a non-dairy option like almond milk to see if your skin improves. Look for products with fewer than 10 grams of sugar per serving.

Try topical antibacterial and retinoids

Dermatologists frequently recommend an acne face wash containing bacteria-killing benzoyl peroxide (3.5 percent strength should be your maximum if you have sensitive skin) and a prescription topical antibiotic such as clindamycin or erythromycin for mild to severe acne. You can use a mild face wash for sensitive skin instead and then apply a benzoyl peroxide acne spot treatment.

Prescription retinoids (such as Retin-A or Tazorac) are "really the standard of treatment for most acne therapy," according to Joshua Zeichner, MD, head of cosmetic and clinical research in dermatology at Mount Sinai Hospital in New York City. Certain medicines, such as Epiduo and Ziana, combine retinoids and antibacterials and may be more effective than the individual components. Retinoids are especially useful for adult acne sufferers since they have anti-wrinkle effects (they help promote collagen synthesis).

Look for salicylic acid

Salicylic acid, which is found in gels, wipes, creams, and face washes, is one of the most popular over-the-counter acne remedies. Salicylic acid decreases swelling and redness while also unclogging pores. To avoid skin from getting overly dry, opt for formulations aimed towards mature women rather than teenagers. To begin, aim for 2% salicylic acid.

Manage your stress

"Stress does not cause skin illness on its own," explains Beth McLellan, MD, director of dermatology at Jacobi Medical Center and researcher at the Montefiore Einstein Center for Cancer Care in New York City.

Researchers aren't sure why stomach-churning worry causes adult acne, but they blame stress chemicals like cortisol for raising inflammation levels in the body and activating oil glands. In any event, reducing stress through exercise, meditation, or whatever approach helps you relax may also help you relax your skin.

Consider blue light therapy

Acne-causing bacteria are killed by blue light beams that enter follicles. In extreme instances, photodynamic treatment combines blue light therapy with a topical medication called Levulan. It is important to note that these treatments may produce temporary redness and are not always reimbursed by insurance. Prices vary considerably based on the location and severity of the acne, but one blue light treatment can cost at least $50 and a photodynamic therapy session can cost $100 or more. The majority of patients will require numerous treatments to achieve good results, although many dermatologists offer package offers.

If you're on a tight budget and suffer from mild to severe adult acne, an at-home device like the Neutrogena Light Therapy Acne Treatment Mask may be a decent option, but it may not be as successful as in-office treatments.

Ask your dermatologist about Aldactone

Prescription Aldactone (spironolactone), which was formerly used to treat high blood pressure, is now finding a second life as a therapy for hormonal acne. The medication (a pill given orally) inhibits androgen receptors, which helps to reduce the testosterone surges that can cause acne in adults.

Pick up tea tree oil

Tea tree oil, which is less irritating than its chemical cousin benzoyl peroxide, has a long history of treating mild to severe acne breakouts. The oil, derived from the leaves of an Australian tree, has antiseptic qualities that aid in the reduction of acne-causing bacteria on the skin and the reduction of inflammation in skin cells.

"We've seen it operate against a wide range of species, including 27 of the 32 acne-causing bacteria strains," says Michael Murray, ND, a naturopath and writer of The Encyclopedia of Natural Medicine. Several studies, including a review of data published in the International Journal of Dermatology, support the plant's potency. Tea tree oil may be found in a range of soaps, skin cleansers, and topical treatments. To see how your skin reacts, look for a minimum concentration of 5% of the oil. If you feel that tea tree is too irritating as an all-over treatment, you may use it as a basic spot treatment for persistent pimples.

Cut back on salt

Some experts believe that sodium has skin effects because iodine, which is often present in table salt and some seafood, may aggravate acne outbreaks. For instance, one 2016 study discovered that acne sufferers consumed substantially more salty meals than an acne-free comparison group.

Stick to low-sodium versions of packaged goods, aim to keep your overall salt consumption under 1,500 mg per day (as recommended by the American Heart Association), and avoid these nutritious items that are deceptively laden with salt.

Pop a birth control pill

According to Dr. Zeichner, oral contraceptives can help balance hormonal surges and control monthly cycles, preventing oil glands from going into overdrive. Doctors can prescribe one of four FDA-approved birth control pill brands for acne treatment: Yaz, Beyaz, Estrostep, and Ortho Tri-Cyclen. Patients using oral contraceptives should be informed of potential birth control side effects such as blood clots or vaginal dryness.

Swap out your daily moisturizer

The skincare products you use on a daily basis can have a significant influence on your complexion. If you have acne, you should not forgo moisturizing, especially if you use drying treatments—however, the type of moisturizer you use can make a difference. "Even acne-prone teens must moisturize to maintain a healthy skin barrier. "Drying acne products and medicines can harm the skin barrier," Arielle Kauvar, MD, head of New York Laser & Skin Care and clinical professor of dermatology at New York University School of Medicine, recently told Prevention.

If you're prone to irritation, stick to oil-free, non-comedogenic, fragrance-free moisturizers. This guarantees that your moisturizer does not clog your pores further or aggravate existing outbreaks.

7

Dr. Sebi's Truth and Myth about Acne

The alkaline diet consists of consuming foods that, when digested, cause your body to produce an alkaline reaction. These foods have a PH of 7 or higher. Alkaline meals are nearly exclusively composed of cleaning vegetables, low sugar fruits, pure water, soups, juices, salads, whole grains, omega oils, and so on, and as such, they give the body and skin all of the nutrients required to sustain health. When following an alkaline diet, it is critical to adhere to the 80/20 rule in order to maintain a healthy bodily balance. This entails eating an alkaline diet that is 80 percent alkaline and 20 percent acidic. This may be a large green salad with a modest quantity of chicken, for example.

How can an Alkaline Diet affect the skin?

Eating alkaline meals helps to relax the body by increasing the PH of the body to an alkaline condition. This aids digestion soothes the system and purifies it. This has the same impact on your skin as the previous method. Alkaline foods are also abundant in vitamins including vitamin A, zinc, protein, and omega 3 fatty acids, which aid in acne treatment. The alkaline diet has also been nicknamed the rosacea diet due to its ability to reduce skin redness. Acidic foods, including artificial sweeteners, coffee, soft drinks, cheese, milk, beer, and so on, cause vascular dilatation and skin flushing. Is it better to start with good or negative news? OK, I'll start with the bad news. The bad news is that any stimulant that wakes you up in the morning by activating your entire body, neurological system, and brain may also activate your sebaceous glands, which can result in acne, rosacea, rosacea papules, flushing, and stress. The good news is that eating an alkaline diet provides you with extra energy! Morning stimulants that create an acidic environment in your body are no longer required.

Should you follow an alkaline diet if you have acne? Why is it important what you consume for your skin?

We'll return to chemistry class for a few minutes to discuss your pH levels and how they connect to your health and skin. The pH of a material indicates whether it is acidic or alkaline. This scale runs from 0 to 14, with 7 representing neutral. If it's above 7, it's alkaline; if it's below 7, it's acidic; as I'll explain later, you want to avoid getting below 7. Too much acid can cause skin eruptions such as acne, eczema, inflammations, and other skin and health problems.

Acid-Alkaline Diet:

The Optimal pH Our beautiful bodies are designed to operate within a very restricted pH range. At 7.365, we want our blood level to be somewhat alkaline. Trouble begins to develop when the blood becomes excessively acidic. Chronic imbalances cause skin eruptions, heartburn, eczema, inflammation, chronic tiredness, irritable bowel syndrome, and even cancer.

Unfortunately, with our Standard American Diet, it is quite simple for our bodies to enter the less-than-ideal acidic zone. Our bodies become a breeding ground for bacteria, yeast, and fungus when we stay in the danger zone. This is related to candida overgrowths, which might be one of the primary causes of your skin problems.

Stop the stress!

Not only does our nutrition influence our pH levels, but if we are regularly stressed, do not exercise, are angry, use prescription and over-the-counter drugs, and smoke, you can be sure we are acidic little women. Our lives can sometimes demand that we go go go without pausing to take a breath. Cortisol and adrenaline, acid-forming chemicals released by stress, flood our bodies.

This isn't good for our beautiful bodies. In addition to lowering our stress levels, eating an acid alkaline diet with a higher alkaline content can help offset some of the stress insanity coursing through us.

Dangers of imbalance:

As a consequence of metabolism, our bodies naturally create acid, but we cannot produce alkaline. So when we overload it with acidic foods like coffee, soda, processed meals, milk, meat, sugar, and bread, to mention a few, it seeks alkaline to balance it out. If it can't get it because we're not eating enough greens, it takes alkaline from our cells, causing those cells to become acidic and disease-prone.

In a nutshell, this imbalance causes problems with our organs and blood, creating an excellent habitat for candida development. As a reminder, this causes toxicity, which manifests itself in the form of acne, eczema, and rashes on our skin.

Foods that make you acidic:

Now that you understand the significance of eating an acid alkaline diet to preserve the delicate pH balance, I'm sure you'd like to know which acidic foods to avoid and which alkaline foods to enjoy. Because it is virtually difficult to eat completely alkaline, a reasonable rule of thumb is to strive for an 80/20 ratio of alkaline to acidic foods.

Alcohol, animal protein, coffee, black tea, soda, energy/sports drinks, processed foods, honey, corn syrup, white & brown sugar, artificial sweeteners, processed soy products, refined grains, white bread, white pasta, table salt, salted nuts, vinegar, soy sauce, and stress are all items to put in your 20% bucket.

Foods that make you Alkaline:

Now comes the fun part! Alkaline water, almonds, Brazil nuts, flax seeds, avocados, garlic, green juices, raw green veggies, lemons, grapefruit, miso, raw tomatoes, root vegetables, seaweed, sprouts, watermelon, moderate amounts of grains: quinoa, wild rice, millet, amaranth, buckwheat, and relaxation should account for 80% of your diet.

Reasons to consume an alkaline diet an acne diet:

Acne is influenced by nutrition and what you eat or do not eat. When the body becomes acidic, it allows yeast, fungi, and bacteria to thrive. Stress causes the production of acid-forming hormones. Therefore, it might have an impact on the body's alkalinity.

The lack of alkaline foods in the Standard American Diet adds to the body's acid-alkaline balance. With all of the acidic things available, such as drinks, processed meals, sugar, and milk, the body craves something alkaline to keep it balanced. When the body consumes acidic meals on a regular basis, it develops a variety of skin issues, including acne, rashes, eczema, psoriasis, and other skin eruptions.

When clients begin to avoid items that are causing havoc in their digestive systems and on their skin, they see a reduction in skin issues. The bumps begin to fade, and the body begins to rebalance. I'm not joking.

Real-life case studies of acne patients who switched to Alkaline Diets

Client #1: Fabulous Massage therapist who ate vegan yet drank a lot of dairy and sweets. I was certain that the pimples on her jawline were caused by her yoga mat. Her skincare products were terrible.

We suggested a basic program that included the Organic Beta Cleanser and the Micro-Crystal Polish. Her acne was causing big blackheads to develop into pustules, and scarring was forming. The skin was considerably improved after peels, extractions, and a series of treatments, but she was still having issues. We repeatedly advised them to avoid sweets and dairy. She cut back on the sweets but kept the dairy. After a trip to Mexico and a yoga retreat where only organic almond milk was offered, the light bulb went out. She raced through the spa door, exclaiming, "Look at my skin! It's shining and perfect!"

Client #2: This customer, a busy executive mom of one, has had skin problems for years. She doesn't need to be persuaded to give up sweets or dairy. She comes in after cheating on a daily basis to exclaim, "two days ago, I drank coffee with sugar and cream, now look at those huge ones." We assist in keeping her skin exfoliated and extracted so that the toxins do not breed additional bacteria in her body.

Don't make these acne treatment mistakes

Teens aren't the only ones that get pimples. Acne can persist long into your 30s, 40s, and beyond. In fact, 15% of adult females suffer from acne. Hormones, stress, and pores blocked by oil, skin cells, and germs are all culprits, just as they were when you were younger.

There are several treatment choices available, ranging from your local drugstore to your dermatologist's clinic. However, you don't want your search for clear skin to cause more harm than good. Make an effort to avoid these typical treatment blunders.

Overdoing washing or scrubbing

Many acne sufferers believe that they must vigorously cleanse their faces. This, however, can irritate the skin, making it more difficult to utilize over-the-counter or prescription acne treatments. Use acne scrubs sparingly since they may aggravate the condition, and avoid cleansers that strip the skin of its natural oils.
"When the skin is dry and irritated, it is more difficult for individuals to take acne medicines, which is ultimately counterproductive," explains Maral Skelsey, MD, head of dermatologic surgery at Georgetown University Medical Center.
"Unless they are perspiring profusely after sports or other activities, most people only need to wash their faces twice daily."
Instead of scrubs and sudsy soaps, use a mild cleanser in the morning and at night.

Squeezing pimples

It may be tempting to burst that zit but resist the urge. It may result in a scar or infection, or it may aggravate your outbreaks. Acne pustules and papules can extend deep into the skin, and pressing them can result in long-term redness and permanent skin depression. "It can also lead to infection and an even bigger pimple in the near term," Skelsey adds. If you can't bear the thought of leaving that pimple alone, apply a warm (not hot) compress to it to help it to heal faster.

Avoiding moisturizer

Acne-prone skin can be dry, especially if retinoids are used to treat it. However, many acne sufferers are hesitant to use moisturizers for fear of exacerbating their breakouts. To keep your skin healthy while treating acne, use a "noncomedogenic" moisturizer. (Non-comedogenic products are those that do not clog pores.)

8

Natural Remedies for Acne that Actually Works

Acne isn't only an adolescent concern for many; it's a condition that lasts into adulthood. Those of us who still have acne-prone skin know that it's a constant fight to not only cure the blemishes that have already appeared on our faces but also to keep them from reappearing, whether by oral medicine or topical treatments that are either prescribed or over-the-counter.

But, when it comes to combating acne, sometimes going back to basics—or going natural—is the best option. We spoke about natural acne treatments with UMA Oils creator Shrankhla Holecek, S.W. Basics founder Adina Grigore, celebrity facialist Joanna Vargas of Joanna Vargas Salon, and board-certified dermatologist Dendy Engelman, MD, FACMS, FAAD.

We asked them which compounds we should look for, what we can create of the natural ingredients we discovered, and why these ingredients are good for acne treatment.

Baking Soda

"Technically, baking soda and water soften blackheads and any clogged pores in the skin," explains Vargas, who adds that baking soda is excellent for congested skin because it is more prone to pore blockages. She suggests making your own baking soda mask and applying it for 10 minutes before applying moisturizer.

Baking soda may also be used to balance the pH of your skin. This is significant since an unbalanced pH can lead to acne outbreaks, dryness, and premature aging.

Apple Cider Vinegar

"It's nature's finest astringent since it helps to balance the pH of the skin, making you less greasy and less dry," explains Grigore of ACV. However, because apple cider vinegar includes acetic acid and alpha-hydroxy acids, it is highly pungent and should be diluted before usage. "I propose a vinegar-to-water ratio of one part vinegar to four parts water. Apply with a cotton ball or a spritzer on your face. There's no need to wash it away, "she claims.

According to Engelman, ACV may also chemically exfoliate the skin, combat blackheads, and reduce hyperpigmentation, "but only when applied appropriately." The chemical "may cause burns and skin irritation, especially if there are any open sores on your skin" if not diluted.

Turmeric

Turmeric is high in antioxidants, which give several skin advantages such as brightening and cleansing the skin. It also contains antimicrobial properties, which "[makes turmeric] ideal for treating eczema, psoriasis, and acne by soothing inflammation and decreasing flare-ups," according to Engelman. Holecek suggests using it with exfoliating bases that are mild on the skin, such as chickpea flour, oat powders, or kaolin clay.

Honey

Because of its antibacterial and humectant qualities, honey is a well-known natural treatment. But, as Engelman points out, not all honey is created equal. Manuka honey, which is produced by honey bees that feed on manuka plants in New Zealand, has the highest antibacterial activity and is excellent for treating acne, inflammation, and skin disorders such as eczema and psoriasis. Honey is also a humectant, which means it retains moisture in the skin once applied, so it leaves the face smooth and moisturized rather than greasy.

Holecek recommends making a mixture with honey, aloe vera, one teaspoon of chickpea flour, and sprinkle turmeric for a DIY facial. Spread the paste on your face, then rinse with cool water and apply an ice cube to the skin for 30 seconds to cure a congested face.

Fine-Grain Salt

"Fine-grain salt cleans thoroughly, eliminates dead skin cells, regulates moisture, and draws toxins from pores, making it especially useful for avoiding acne or treating flare-ups on the face and body," explains Grigore. Sea salt may also aid in the treatment of skin diseases such as eczema, psoriasis, acne, and even wounds due to its antimicrobial qualities. "To use sea salt, moisten your face or body, put some salt on your wet palm, so it adheres, and then gently apply it over your skin. You may either let it for a few minutes or quickly rinse it. Just be careful not to scrub too hard since it is extremely abrasive on its own."

Tea Tree Oil

According to specialists, tea tree oil is an excellent antibacterial and anti-inflammatory agent. "It's well-known for its antibacterial, antibiotic, and antifungal qualities, making it a simple and efficient spot treatment," Grigore says.

According to Engelman, "it decreases redness and swelling of the skin while also decreasing acne outbreaks and eliminating dandruff-causing fungus."

Grigore recommends diluting tea tree oil with extra virgin olive oil or organic jojoba oil and applying it straight on a zit.

9

Dr. Sebi Approved Herbs and Supplements to Fighting Acne

A cne is caused by blocked pores and germs, and it can be difficult to treat. Over-the-counter and prescription medications may be helpful, but some can have significant adverse effects. If standard therapies fail, or if you wish to try something more natural, you may want to consider herbal remedies.

Long before contemporary therapies, herbal medicines were utilized to treat acne and other skin problems. Despite the paucity of data on many herbal remedies, anecdotal evidence abounds.

Herbal therapies are less likely to have adverse effects than contemporary medications. Herbs with antibacterial, anti-inflammatory, and antiseptic effects are available. These characteristics may aid in the reduction of acne-causing bacteria and inflammation, as well as the healing of blemishes.

According to Researchers

Manjistha

Manjistha (Rubia cordifolia) is a perennial plant that is commonly used in Ayurvedic medicine. It is considered to help your lymphatic system, which is important for good skin. According to studies, manjistha contains anti-inflammatory, antibacterial, and antiandrogenic properties that may aid in the prevention and treatment of acne.

Neem

Another well-known Ayurvedic herb is neem (Azadirachta indica). According to a 2010 research, neem oil includes the following compounds:

- Antibacterial
- Antifungal
- Antiseptic
- Antioxidant
- Anti-inflammatory

Neem has traditionally been used to treat skin problems such as acne, eczema, and psoriasis. A 2001 research found that neem had antibacterial action against a variety of microorganisms. This contains Staphylococcus aureus, a bacteria associated with acne.

Tea tree

The tea tree (melaleuca alternifolia) is a plant that is used to heal skin conditions and wounds. It possesses antibacterial and anti-inflammatory properties that may help to reduce the number of acne lesions. A topical gel containing 5% tea tree oil was compared to a topical cream containing 5% benzoyl peroxide in a 1990 research. Both treatments decreased the number of acne lesions, both inflamed and noninflamed. Although tea tree oil took longer to function, it had fewer negative effects. Dryness, itching, inflammation, and redness were among them.

Witch hazel and other herbs

Astringent tannins in witch hazel may help cure acne by eliminating excess skin oil. It also has anti-inflammatory properties and can be used to decrease redness and bruises. Witch hazel is frequently used on its own or as a foundation for DIY acne treatments.

Other antibacterial and anti-inflammatory herbs that may aid in acne healing include:

- Calendula
- Chamomile
- Lavender
- Rosemary

Basil

According to the specialists at Little Barn Apothecary, the green herb is a lot superior astringent than alcohol (or those harsh acne treatments like benzoyl peroxide). "[Basil] aids in the removal of impurities from the skin and works as an antibacterial," Scoggins says. "It will assist with any inflammation that is frequently linked with acne skin, as well as control oil production, which is a cause of certain outbreaks." Don't have anything with basil in it? According to Scoggins, you may make your own cleaning mask by mashing up a few stems and smearing them on your face.

Geranium

Look for a geranium in your skin-care products if your breakouts are blackheads. Scoggins claims that "geranium oil helps to slow down the symptoms of aging and control your oil production." This is critical because, as he says, blackheads "appear when there is an overproduction of oil and blocked pores."

Blue yarrow

This beautiful plant isn't as fragile as it looks in the wild. "Blue yarrow is a very strong astringent that can help with skin healing, and it's also one of those extremely antiseptic herbs that will clear skin of germs and prevent breakouts," adds Scoggins. "It's fantastic for irritated skin and blackheads," says the author. Reach for it when your skin is on the verge of exploding.

Hibiscus

Are you looking to add some anti-aging to your skin-care routine? Consider this flowery stunner. "Hibiscus has been dubbed nature's Botox," Morgan explains. "It's also excellent for cleaning and firming the skin. It aids in the reduction of fine lines and the appearance of wrinkles." In other words, it's beautiful yet potent.

Supplemental Components that Fight Acne

L-Carnitine: This is an amino acid that can assist in decreasing excessive oil production in the skin. Oily skin types may have pores that clog more easily, resulting in pimples and blackheads. L-carnitine will assist in reducing excessive oil production, giving your skin a healthy shine without making it seem greasy.

Pantetheine: This vitamin B5 derivative aids the body's metabolization of oils, preventing excessive oil excretion into the skin. While some oil is necessary to keep your skin naturally hydrated, too much oil may clog your pores and leave you looking glossy and greasy, especially on the forehead, nose, and chin (the T-zone). Pantetheine can aid in the equilibrium of skin oils.

And now for some of Traditional Chinese Medicine's best-kept secrets.

Oldenlandia: This addresses the root cause of acne by removing harmful heat that can promote inflammation. It also has powerful antibacterial, radical-scavenging, and antioxidant capabilities that will aid in the battle against acne-causing bacteria in the skin.

Gardenia Seeds: Gardenia seed components assist in combating inflammation, which causes skin blemishes to seem red and irritated. According to TCM, they assist in discharging internal fire that might appear on the skin. These properties aid in the restoration of an even skin tone.

Pimples can be caused by specific types of bacteria being stuck in pores, according to Moutan Root Bark. This herb has been shown to kill germs and scavenge toxins, therefore combating acne's root cause. Moutan Root Bark, according to TCM, aids in blood cooling.

Red Peony Root: This plant has powerful antifungal qualities and aids in the movement of blood and the removal of blood heat. According to TCM, blood heat can show itself as skin irritation.

Bupleurum, also known as Chai Hu, has long been known to have anti-inflammatory properties. Because inflammation is one of the causes of acne lesions appearing red and larger, it is important to boost the body's capacity to combat inflammation in order to improve the skin's look. According to TCM, Chai Hu also enhances the operation of the liver meridian system, which is directly connected to skin problems.

Skullcap Root: This root aids in the removal of moist heat from the body. It also fights germs that may be causing acne and aids in the scavenging of harmful free radicals.

How to use herbs for acne

Using a cotton swab or cotton ball, apply witch hazel straight to your skin. It can also be used in conjunction with carrier oil and other acne herbal treatments. Witch hazel should not be consumed or injected.

Witch hazel may be used as part of your skincare routine to remove makeup, clean, and refresh your skin.

The Farmer's Almanac advises the following methods for making your own witch hazel decoction for the greatest results:

- In a big stainless steel saucepan, combine the witch hazel bark and twigs.
- Cover with distilled water.
- Bring to a boil and reduce to low heat for at least 30 minutes.
- Cool overnight.
- Strain decoction and pour into a glass jar.
- Store in the refrigerator.

Before using neem oil, dilute it with water or carrier oil such as coconut oil or olive oil. Neem oil soap is an excellent way to get acquainted with the herb. It should be available at your local natural health store. Be aware that neem oil has a strong odor that many people dislike.

Manjistha powder is frequently mixed with other plants such as neem. It's also in capsules and soap.

10

What Type of Foods are Believed to Improve Your Acne?

Consuming low-glycemic meals high in complex carbs may lower your chances of acquiring acne. The following foods include complex carbohydrates:

- Whole grains
- Legumes
- Unprocessed fruits and vegetables

Foods containing the following components are also considered to be helpful to the skin due to their ability to decrease inflammation:

- The mineral zinc
- Vitamin a and e
- Chemicals called antioxidants

Some skin-friendly food choices include:

- Yellow and orange fruits and vegetables include carrots, apricots, and sweet potatoes.
- Spinach, as well as other dark green and leafy veggies.
- Tomatoes
- Blueberries
- Turkey
- Pumpkin seeds
- Beans, peas, and lentils
- Salmon, mackerel, and other kinds of fatty fish

- Nuts
- Whole-wheat bread
- Brown rice
- Quinoa

Everyone's body is unique, and some people experience more acne when they eat specific foods. Experimenting with your diet under the guidance of your doctor might be beneficial in determining what works best for you.

When planning your diet, keep in mind any dietary allergies or sensitivities you may have.

Are there any studies that indicate that these meals are beneficial to your skin?

Low-glycemic diets

Several recent studies show that eating a low-glycemic diet, or one low in simple sugars can help to prevent and treat acne. In one study of Korean patients, researchers discovered that maintaining a low-glycemic load for 10 weeks can lead to considerable improvements in acne.

Another study published in the Journal of the American Academy of Dermatology discovered that following a low-glycemic, high-protein diet for 12 weeks reduced acne in males while also resulting in weight reduction.

Zinc

Consuming zinc-rich foods may also help prevent and cure acne, according to research. Zinc-rich foods include the following:
- Pumpkin seeds
- Cashews
- Beef
- Turkey

- Quinoa
- Lentils
- Seafood such as oysters and crab

Researchers looked at the link between zinc levels in the blood and acne severity in one study published in the BioMed Research International Journal. Zinc is a dietary mineral that is essential for skin growth as well as metabolism and hormone levels.

The researchers discovered that low zinc levels were associated with more severe acne occurrences. To treat patients with severe acne, they recommend increasing the quantity of zinc in the diet to 40 milligrams per day. According to research, even those who do not have acne should consume the same quantity of zinc.

Vitamins A and E

Researchers discovered that low levels of vitamins A and E appear to be connected to severe instances of acne in a study published in the Journal of Cutaneous and Ocular Toxicology.

They believe that by increasing their intake of foods containing these vitamins, acne sufferers may be able to reduce the severity of their acne. Before using vitamin A pills, see your doctor. Toxic levels of vitamin A can permanently harm your main organs.

Antioxidants and omega-3 fatty acids

Omega-3 fatty acids are present in plants and animal protein sources such as fish and eggs. Antioxidants are molecules that bind to and neutralize harmful poisons in the body. Omega-3 fatty acids and antioxidants are considered to work together to decrease inflammation.

studies have found a link between an increase in omega-3 and antioxidant consumption and a decrease in acne.

According to research published in the journal Lipids in Health and Disease, participants who took a daily omega-3 and antioxidant supplement were able to minimize their acne as well as enhance their mental health.

Because acne frequently causes mental discomfort, omega-3 and antioxidant intake may be quite useful to those suffering from the illness.

DO'S AND DON'T'S OF ACNE PREVENTION DIET

There are so many things you wish you could forget about your adolescence - but you just can't seem to get rid of the pimples. Adult acne is on the rise, according to the American Academy of Dermatology (AAD), and 15% of women have outbreaks.

Why is frequently a puzzle for doctors to solve — and it involves more than simply buying a nice benzoyl peroxide lotion at the supermarket like you did when you were 17. Some specialists believe that what you consume may have a role in pimple production, although they do not all agree.

While some foods, such as dairy, sugar, and processed meals like potato chips, crackers, and granola bars, are suspected of causing acne, "research is not conclusive on what foods cause acne." We do know, however, that our skin reacts differently from person to person," says Gretchen Frieling, MD, a board-certified dermatopathologist in Boston. "It is likely that various meals will have different impacts on different people," she explains.

According to Dr. Frieling, your food can impact sebum (oil) production in the skin, hormone control, and inflammation, all of which can set the scene for acne. But it's not just about diet. Acne development is multifaceted. According to a study published in the journal Clinical, Cosmetic, and Investigational Dermatology in December 2017, emotional stress is one factor that contributes to more severe breakouts, probably because stress causes sebaceous (oil-producing) glands to go into overdrive. "While stress is not the only cause of pimples, it certainly exacerbates acne-prone skin," Frieling adds.

To discover a clear skin solution that works for you, it's vital to look at your entire body — food, skin-care routines, topical treatments (specifically, ensuring sure they're anti-comedogenic, so they don't clog pores). "Some acne-causing variables, such as genetics and skin type, are beyond your control. "However, what you eat can have a significant impact on your general skin health and sebum production," adds Frieling.

In short, research published in April 2016 in Dermatology Practical & Conceptual, 71% of acne study participants sought to modify their diet to address their skin issues, but they frequently missed out on items (particularly refined carbs) that have some of the strongest hypothesized ties to acne. Identifying your personal triggers may need some self-experimentation. The AAD suggests paying attention to your breakouts and asking yourself if specific meals appear to aggravate them and whether they improve when you avoid certain foods.

Here are some items to keep an eye out for, as well as tips on how to construct an overall diet that will keep outbreaks away.

Don't eat refined carbs or meals with a high glycemic index.

According to Whitney P. Bowe, MD, a clinical assistant professor of dermatology at the Icahn School of Medicine at Mount Sinai Medical Center in New York City and Medical Director of Integrative Dermatology, Aesthetics, and Wellness at Advanced Dermatology in Briarcliff Manor, New York, some of the strongest evidence to date links high-GI foods to acne.

According to Harvard Health Publishing, refined carbohydrates and sugars like white bread, russet potatoes, boxed macaroni and cheese, and other highly processed foods have a high GI. According to the AAD, this increase in blood sugar levels creates a cascade of reactions that raises inflammation and leads the skin to produce more oil and clog the pores, which lays the scene for acne. "You want to avoid anything white or polished," adds Dr. Bowe. Change from white bread to whole-grain bread and from white rice to brown rice. According to Harvard, these foods (100 percent whole-wheat bread and brown rice) are lower on the glycemic index; they're not only less processed, but they're also richer in fiber, which slows the increase of blood sugar after a meal.

Do: Choose fish and other healthy fat-rich foods

Focusing on an anti-inflammatory diet may help to soothe breakout-prone skin. "Because acne is an inflammatory illness in and of itself," explains Frieling, "foods that induce inflammation add to the pathophysiology of acne." Furthermore, persistent inflammation can cause the breakdown of elastin and collagen fibers in the skin, aggravating wrinkles, according to a study published in the journal Cell Transplant in May 2018. (According to the Cleveland Clinic, collagen is a protein found throughout the body, including muscles, bones, and skin.) She goes on to say that worsening acne (more red or painful lesions), drooping, or loss of smoothness are all signs of persistent inflammation.

While bad fat might cause inflammation, "you don't want to avoid fat entirely," adds Bowe. "You want to consume good fats, such as omega-3 fatty acids." According to the National Institutes of Health, healthy fats include omega-3 fatty acid-rich foods like salmon and sardines, as well as flaxseed, walnuts, and chia seeds. Unhealthy fats include artificial trans fats, which were formally prohibited in 2018 by the US Food and Drug Administration, according to a June 2018 Washington Post story. According to Harvard Medical School, you should also avoid eating too many saturated fats. Full-fat dairy, fast food, and commercially baked products are all sources of harmful fats, according to the researchers.

Don't: Consume excessive amounts of milk and other dairy products

According to the AAD, several studies have found a relationship between ingesting milk and other dairy products and an increased risk of acne. There are two possible explanations: These foods cause the body to release insulin and growth hormones, which lead to breakouts.

According to an analysis of 14 research published in the journal Nutrients in August 2018, consuming any dairy was related to a 25% higher risk of acne in children and young people aged 7 to 30, compared to not eating any dairy at all.

"Milk proteins, particularly casein and whey, are emerging as culprits in the acne relationship," adds Bowe. "However, milk contains hormones that are precursors to testosterone, and this, coupled with protein, maybe a combination that causes acne. We continued finding a greater relationship between skim milk and acne at first, and we still don't know why it's stronger than for whole milk."

One person may be able to tolerate dairy well, but another may get breakouts as a result of a dairy-rich diet. "Our systems' reactions to these hormones may differ from person to person, but dairy increases an insulin-like hormone called IGF-1, which can contribute to breakouts," Frieling says, echoing the findings of the Nutrients analysis.

If acne is an issue, Bowe suggests looking for non-dairy options, such as calcium-fortified soy and almond milk. They will almost certainly be fortified with vitamin D, which is a plus because some research, such as a study published in the journal Dermato-

Endocrinology in February 2018, has suggested that a vitamin D deficiency may be linked to acne, possibly because an adequate amount of vitamin D quells inflammation.

Do: Consume a variety of heart-healthy and skin-friendly nuts.

Many nuts, such as walnuts and almonds, are high in omega-3 fatty acids, which can help reduce inflammation, as well as zinc. According to a review published in the journal Dermatology Research and Practice in July 2014, zinc is anti-inflammatory, lowers levels of the bacteria that causes acne (Cutibacterium acnes), and may help reduce sebum production. Bowe claims that nutrient-containing lotions and supplements have been used topically to cure acne. "I try to encourage obtaining it through food or taking a multivitamin because pills might cause nausea," she says.

Don't: Overindulge in the chocolate milk (and Do Be Wary of Chocolate Itself)

The true link between chocolate milk and acne, like all dairy, is debatable and requires additional investigation. However, early research published in the 1960s and 1970s showed that milk chocolate was associated with acne. That study did not precisely look at which component of milk chocolate — sugar, nonfat milk solids, milk fat, or cocoa — was responsible for acne, and while this is debatable, some later research suggests there is a relationship.

For example, very small research published in May 2014 in The Journal of Clinical and Aesthetic Dermatology discovered that ingesting 100 percent cocoa was related to worsened acne in acne-prone men. Further research published in the Journal of the American Academy of Dermatology in July 2016 examined the impact of consuming chocolate vs. jelly beans. After 48 hours, the chocolate group had roughly five more acne lesions than the jelly bean group, which had fewer than one.

While the case isn't closed on whether chocolate alone causes acne, Bowe suggests avoiding it for those who are acne-prone due to the milk and sugar levels of milk chocolate.

Do: Eat antioxidant-rich fruits and vegetables on your plate

Antioxidants, which are also renowned for their anti-inflammatory effects, can help with acne. Antioxidants are found in vividly colored fruits and vegetables, such as peppers, spinach, and berries, according to the National Center for Complementary and Integrative Health. Furthermore, consuming nutritious foods strong in antioxidants can help the body combat free radicals and oxidative stress, which Bowe claims can help with acne. (The AAD describes free radicals as "molecules that cause skin damage and aging," whereas oxidative stress happens when there are more free radicals present than antioxidants to fight them, according to an article published in January 2014 in the Asian Pacific Journal of Cancer Prevention.)

According to Frieling, a diet rich in fruits and vegetables offers "vitamins and minerals that reduce inflammation, such as zinc, vitamin A, and vitamin E." Among the nutrient-dense foods she recommends are carrots, pumpkin, squash, beans, spinach, kale, sunflower seeds, broccoli, and brown rice.

Don't: Go overboard on eating fried foods

For your health, you should minimize harmfully saturated and trans fats, such as those found in fried meals and processed baked products. These promote inflammation in the body, but "oily, fatty meals are not what causes acne," according to Frieling. (If you cook with a lot of oil all the time, she explains, you could get oil on your skin, which could clog pores, but that's completely another issue.)

"While most physicians and nutritionists would advise against consuming these items for your general health, they are not what would clean up your skin," Frieling explains.

Do: Consume probiotic-rich foods such as yogurt.

"Probiotics are quite popular right now when it comes to acne," adds Bowe. Probiotics, or good bacteria, are microorganisms that are considered to have positive effects on the gut, according to the Mayo Clinic. According to an article published in the International Journal of Women's Dermatology in April 2015, these beneficial bugs may reduce inflammation to help prevent acne, and when added to the fermentation process (to turn milk into yogurt), they may also decrease levels of the growth factor found in milk, called IGF-1. As a result, yogurt may be one form of dairy that may be used as part of an anti-acne diet.

While further study is needed, probiotics' function in clean skin appears promising. According to the Mayo Clinic, probiotics may be found in yogurt containing live active cultures, sauerkraut, kefir, and kimchi, as well as supplements.

Although additional research is needed to establish that probiotics are good meals for clean skin, Bowe believes that they may produce a better bacterial ecology in the stomach, which may help avoid the chain of events that leads to inflammation and acne. Frieling also suggests eating probiotic-rich meals to help clear up acne. She recommends including kimchi, yogurt, sauerkraut, miso, tempeh, and kombucha into your diet.

11

Powerful Home Remedies for Acne

Acne is one of the most common skin disorders, affecting up to 85% of young people worldwide.

Traditional acne treatments like salicylic acid, niacinamide, and benzoyl peroxide have been proven to be the most effective, but they may be expensive and have undesirable side effects, including dryness, redness, and irritation.

This has caused many individuals to search for natural acne cures at home. According to one research, 77 percent of acne sufferers have attempted alternative acne treatments. Many home treatments lack scientific support, and further study on their efficacy is required. However, if you are seeking alternative therapies, there are still alternatives available to you.

The most effective acne treatments are standard clinical procedures. You can also attempt home remedies. However, further study on their efficacy is required.

Here are a few acne home treatments:
1. Apply apple cider vinegar

Fermenting apple cider or the unfiltered liquid from crushed apples yields apple cider vinegar. It, like other vinegar, is well-known for its ability to combat a wide range of germs and fungi.
Organic acids, like citric acid, present in apple cider vinegar have been shown to destroy acnes.

Succinic acid, another organic acid, has been demonstrated in studies to reduce inflammation produced by P. acnes, perhaps preventing scarring. Lactic acid, another acid found in apple cider vinegar, may also help to fade acne scars.

While some components of apple cider vinegar may be beneficial for acne, there is presently no evidence to support its usage for this reason. Some dermatologists advise avoiding using apple cider vinegar at all since it might cause skin irritation.

How to use it
- Combine one part apple cider vinegar and three parts water (use more water for sensitive skin).
- Using a cotton ball, gently apply the mixture to the skin after cleaning.
- Allow for 5–20 seconds before rinsing with water and patting dry.
- Repeat this method 1–2 times each day, if necessary.

It is crucial to know that using apple cider vinegar on your skin might result in burns and irritation. If you decide to give it a shot, start with a tiny quantity and dilute it with water.

Apple cider vinegar's organic acids may aid in the killing of acne-causing bacteria and the reduction of scarring. It should be used with caution since it can cause burns or irritation when applied to the skin.

2. Take a zinc supplement
Zinc is a mineral that is necessary for cell development, hormone synthesis, metabolism, and immunological function.

In comparison to other natural acne remedies, it has received very little research.

According to research, persons with acne have lower zinc levels in their blood than those with clean skin. Taking zinc orally may also help decrease acne, according to many studies.

A 2014 study, for example, discovered that zinc is more successful at treating severe and inflammatory acne than in treating mild acne.

Although the ideal zinc dose for acne has not been determined, numerous earlier research has found that 30–45 mg of elemental zinc per day results in a substantial decrease in acne.

The elemental zinc content of a chemical is its amount of zinc. Zinc is accessible in a variety of forms, each of which contains different quantities of elemental zinc. At 80 percent, zinc oxide has the most elemental zinc.

The suggested safe upper limit for zinc is 40 mg per day, so unless you're under the guidance of a medical practitioner, it's generally better not to exceed that quantity. Taking too much zinc may result in side effects such as stomach discomfort and gut inflammation.

It's also worth mentioning that applying zinc directly to the skin hasn't been shown to be effective. This may be related to the fact that zinc does not absorb well through the skin. Acne sufferers have lower zinc levels than those with clean skin. Several research indicates that consuming zinc orally may help to decrease acne.

3. Make a honey and cinnamon mask

Honey and cinnamon have the potential to combat germs and decrease inflammation, both of which contribute to acne.

According to a 2017 study, the combination of honey and cinnamon bark extract has antibacterial properties against P. acnes.

According to other studies, honey can inhibit or stop the growth of P. acnes on its own. This discovery, however, does not necessarily imply that honey is a good acne treatment.

A study of 136 acne sufferers discovered that adding honey to the skin after using antibacterial soap was no more helpful at curing acne than using the soap alone. While honey and cinnamon's anti-inflammatory and antibacterial qualities may help with acne, further study is needed.

How to create a honey-cinnamon face mask
- Combine two tablespoons of honey and 1 teaspoon cinnamon to make a paste.
- After washing your face, apply the mask and let it on for 10–15 minutes.
- Rinse the mask well and wipe your face dry.

Honey and cinnamon are both anti-inflammatory and antimicrobial. They may help to decrease acne, but further research is needed.

4. Spot treat with tea tree oil
Tea tree oil is an essential oil derived from the leaves of Melaleuca alternifolia, a tiny Australian tree.
It has a well-known capacity to combat germs and decrease skin irritation.

Furthermore, numerous studies have discovered that using tea tree oil to the skin may help to decrease acne.
Another small research discovered that, as compared to benzoyl peroxide, participants who used a tea tree oil ointment for acne had less dry skin and discomfort. They were also happy with the therapy.

Given that long-term use of topical and oral antibiotics for acne might lead to bacterial resistance, tea tree oil may be a useful alternative. Because tea tree oil is quite powerful, it should always be diluted before putting it on your skin.

How to use it
- Combine 1 part tea tree oil and 9 parts water.
- Dip a cotton swab into the solution and dab it on the afflicted regions.
- If desired, apply moisturizer.
- Repeat this method 1–2 times each day, if necessary.

Tea tree oil is anti-bacterial and anti-inflammatory in nature. Acne may be reduced by applying it to the skin.

5. Apply green tea to your skin

Green tea has a lot of antioxidants, so drinking it can help you stay healthy. It may also aid in the reduction of acne. This is most likely due to the polyphenols in green tea, which help combat germs and decrease inflammation, both of which are major causes of acne. There hasn't been much study into the advantages of drinking green tea for acne, and further research is needed.

In a small study, 80 women were given 1,500 mg of green tea extract every day for four weeks. By the end of the study, women who took the extract had less acne on their noses, chins, and around their lips.

According to research, consuming green tea may reduce blood sugar and insulin levels, both of which can contribute to the development of acne.

Several studies have also found that using green tea straight to the skin may assist with acne. According to studies, the primary antioxidant in green tea, epigallocatechin-3-gallate (EGCG), lowers sebum production, fights inflammation, and inhibits the growth of P. acnes in acne-prone individuals.

Several studies have indicated that applying green tea extract to the skin decreases sebum production and pimples in acne sufferers.

Green tea creams and lotions are available for buy, but making your own at home is just as easy.

How to use it
- Steep green tea for 3–4 minutes in boiling water.
- Set aside the tea to cool.
- Apply the tea to your skin with a cotton ball or spritz it on using a spray bottle.
- Allow it to dry before rinsing with water and patting your skin dry.
- You may also construct a mask with the remaining tea leaves and honey.

Green tea is strong in antioxidants, which aid in the battle against germs and inflammation. According to certain studies, using green tea extract to the skin may help decrease acne.

6. Apply witch hazel
Witch hazel is made from the bark and leaves of the North American witch hazel plant Hamamelis virginiana. It includes tannins, which are naturally antimicrobial and anti-inflammatory.
As a result, it is used to treat a wide variety of skin conditions, including dandruff, eczema, varicose veins, burns, bruises, insect bites, and acne.

Currently, there seems to be a very little study on witch hazel's potential to cure acne. A skincare business financed a small trial in which 30 people with mild to severe acne received a three-step face treatment twice daily for six weeks.

One of the components in the second phase of the therapy was witch hazel. The majority of people had shown significant improvement in their acne at the conclusion of the study. Witch hazel may also help to fight bacteria while also reducing skin irritation and inflammation, which may both contribute to acne.

How to use it
- In a small saucepan, combine 1 tablespoon witch hazel bark and 1 cup water.
- Soak the witch hazel in water for 30 minutes before bringing it to a boil on the burner.
- Reduce to low heat and simmer, covered, for 10 minutes.
- Take the pan off the heat and set it aside for 10 minutes.
- Strain the liquid and store it in a well-sealed jar.
- Apply with a cotton ball to clean skin 1–2 times per day or as needed.

It is essential to remember that commercially produced versions may lack tannins since they are frequently lost during the distillation process. Applying witch hazel to the skin may help to alleviate irritation and inflammation. It may be useful for acne sufferers, but further study is needed.

7. Use aloe vera to moisturize

Aloe vera is a tropical plant whose leaves generate a clear gel. Lotions, creams, ointments, and soaps often include the gel.
It's often used to treat abrasions, rashes, burns, and other skin issues. Aloe vera gel, when applied to the skin, may help with wound healing, burn therapy, and inflammation reduction.

Salicylic acid and sulfur, both of which are widely utilized in the treatment of acne, are found in aloe vera. Salicylic acid applied to the skin reduces acne, according to studies.

Several studies have also suggested that aloe vera gel, when coupled with other ingredients such as tretinoin cream or tea tree oil, may help with acne. While research indicates promise, the anti-acne effects of aloe vera deserve more scientific investigation.

How to use it
- Using a spoon, scrape the gel off the aloe plant.
- As a moisturizer, apply the gel straight to clean skin.
- Do this 1–2 times each day, or as needed.

You may also purchase aloe vera gel from a shop, but make sure it is pure aloe with no additional chemicals. When applied to the skin, aloe vera gel can aid in the healing of wounds, the treatment of burns, and the reduction of inflammation. It may be useful for acne sufferers, but further study is needed.

8. Reduce stress

The relationship between stress and acne is not completely understood. Hormones generated during stressful times may boost sebum production and inflammation, exacerbating acne.

Stress may also have an impact on gut flora and create inflammation throughout the body, which may be connected to acne. Furthermore, stress has been shown to delay wound healing, which may slow the healing of acne lesions.

Several studies have identified a link between stress and acne. However, because each of these trials was tiny, additional study is required. One study with 80 individuals discovered no link between stress severity and acne. It was found, however, that the severity of acne may be connected to people's capacity to manage stress. Certain relaxation and stress-reduction therapies may help with acne, but further study is needed.

Ways to reduce stress
- Practice yoga
- Meditate
- Take deep breaths
- Get more sleep
- Engage in physical activity

Hormones generated during times of stress may aggravate acne. Stress reduction may aid in the treatment of acne.

9. Exercise regularly

There hasn't been a lot of research done on the effects of exercise on acne. Nonetheless, exercise influences body systems in ways that may aid in acne treatment. Exercise, for example, aids in the circulation of blood. Increased blood flow to the skin nourishes the cells, which may aid in acne prevention and healing.

Exercise also affects hormone levels and regulation.

Exercise has been shown in many studies to help decrease stress and anxiety, both of which may contribute to the development of acne. According to the US Department of Health and Human Services, adults should get 150 minutes of aerobic exercise per week and two days of strength training each week.

Walking, hiking, jogging, and weightlifting are all examples of this. Exercise has an impact on several factors that may help with acne. These include promoting healthy blood circulation and assisting in stress reduction.

12

Dr. Sebi Alkaline Diet

What is the Dr. Sebi diet all about?

The plant-based diet is a type of alkaline diet that was created to assist cells to heal themselves by combining a limited food with supplements.

"Dr." Sebi, whose actual name is Alfredo Darrington Bowman, was born in Honduras in 1933. He was not a medical nor a non-medical doctor, nor was he a licensed healthcare practitioner of any sort (though his site calls him a "pathologist, herbalist, biochemist, and naturalist"). Alfredo was jailed for practicing medicine without a license after being involved in a number of civil and criminal lawsuits throughout his life. Bowman died in August of this year.

Throughout his life, his diet attracted a lot of famous supporters, including Michael Jackson, but it was also fraught with controversy. He was known to dispute that HIV causes AIDS and was actually sued by New York state in 1993 after claiming to have "fixed AIDS." He was ordered to avoid making medical claims regarding the benefits of his diet.

The diet proposes a strict vegan diet and is based on the idea that all illnesses are caused by a localized failure of the body's mucous membranes. Bowman suggested that by generating an alkaline atmosphere, illnesses might be eradicated.

There is a "Nutritional Guide" as part of Bowman's diet, which gives a list of items you're permitted to eat (it's specific), as well as some additional rules.

Dr. Sebi's "Cell Food" supplements are also recommended in his diet. The program, which has gender-specific choices, costs between $750 and $1,500.

Rules of the diet (per Dr Sebi):
1. If the food is not on his "list of foods," it is not advised.
2. Drink one gallon of pure spring water every day.
3. Strict attention to the "food list and guidance" yields the greatest outcomes for "disease reversal."
4. No animal products, hybrid foods, canned fruits, seedless fruits, or alcohol may be eaten.
5. According to Sebi, using the microwave can "destroy your food," therefore avoid using it.

1. What does it mean to alkalize the body?

An alkaline diet is based on the idea that the foods you consume may help you manage your body's pH. Because the nutrients we eat produce metabolic waste, the waste is said to have a pH ranging from alkaline to acidic.

To support distinct physiological activities, the human body has varied pH values in different regions, with organs like the stomach being more acidic and blood being more alkaline. pH homeostasis in many organs and fluids is closely controlled.

Our bodies have built-in acid-base balance via the lungs, kidneys, and buffer systems via complicated excretion and reabsorption mechanisms. Urine is one of the body products that is directly influenced by the food and fluids we eat. This is an example of a kidney-controlled system for controlling blood pH.

Do alkaline diets work?

The Dr. Sebi diet is one of many "alkaline diets" centered on the issue of metabolic waste. The components of these diets are typically healthy enough in that they encourage eating more nutritious plant-based foods, which would benefit almost everyone. Meats, shellfish, eggs, dairy, sugar, processed foods, and wheat are commonly criticized or eliminated from an alkaline diet.

While these dietary adjustments would undoubtedly enhance many people's health (by reduced sugar and calorie intake, as well as increased fiber and fruit and vegetable intake), the concept that food patterns or components may substantially alter our strong, built-in acid-base balance is unscientific.

There is no study behind alkalinizing the body, and science does not back the promises claimed by Bowman or similar alkaline regimens. Many research on alkaline diets have been evaluated and meta-analyzed and the findings are in: neither the alkaline diet nor its associated "acid-ash hypothesis" has been demonstrated to prevent or reduce illness. To mention a few, this lack of effect includes bone health and osteoporosis, cancer, and glucose and insulin responses.

Dr. Sebi food list

And if you're curious, here's the complete list of foods allowed on the Dr. Sebi diet:

Vegetables
- Amaranth greens
- Avocado
- Bell Peppers
- Chayote (a Mexican squash)
- Sea vegetables
- Squash
- Tomatoes (only cherry or plum varieties)
- Purslane (verdolaga)
- Wild arugula

- Cucumber
- Dandelion greens
- Garbanzo beans
- Izote (Cactus flowers/leaves)
- Kale
- Lettuce (but not iceberg)
- Mushrooms (but not shiitake)
- Nopales (Mexican cactus)
- Okra
- Olives
- Onions
- Tomatillos
- Turnip greens
- Zucchini
- Watercress

Fruits
- Figs
- Grapes (if needed)
- Limes
- Mango
- Melons (if needed)
- Orange (Seville or sour is best)
- Papayas
- Peaches
- Apples
- Bananas
- Berries (but not cranberries)
- Elderberries
- Cantaloupe
- Cherries
- Currants

- Dates
- Pears
- Plums
- Prickly pear (cactus fruit)
- Prunes
- Raisins (if needed)
- Young coconuts
- Soursops (if you can find them)
- Tamarind

Grains
- Quinoa
- Rye
- Amaranth
- Fonio
- Kamut
- Spelled
- Tef
- Wild rice

Oils
- Sesame oil
- Hempseed oil
- Avocado oil
- Olive oil (only uncooked)
- Coconut oil (only uncooked)
- Grapeseed oil

Nuts and seeds
- Raw tahini
- Walnuts
- Brazil nuts

- Hemp seeds
- Raw sesame seeds

Seasonings
- Achiote
- Cayenne Thyme Powdered seaweeds
- Pure agave syrup
- Date sugar
- Onion powder
- Habanero
- Sage
- Pure sea salt
- Basil
- Bay leaf
- Cloves
- Dill
- Savory
- Sweet basil
- Tarragon

Teas
- Fennel
- Ginger
- Raspberry
- Burdock
- Chamomile
- Elderberry
- Tila

Alkaline diet and blood PH

An alkaline diet is one that is designed to help balance the pH of the fluids in your body, such as your blood and urine.

This diet is also known as the alkaline ash diet, alkaline acid diet, acid ash diet, pH diet, and Dr. Sebi's alkaline diet (Dr. Sebi was an herbalist who created a plant-based version of the diet).

The mineral density of the meals you eat contributes to your pH. All living creatures and life forms on Earth rely on maintaining proper pH levels, and it is commonly stated that sickness and disorder cannot take root in a body with a balanced pH.

The ideas of the acid ash theory contribute to the alkaline diet's tenets. According to a study published in the Journal of Bone and Mineral Research, "the acid-ash hypothesis proposes that protein and grain foods, combined with a low potassium intake, produce a diet acid load, net acid excretion (NAE), increased urine calcium, and calcium release from the skeleton, leading to osteoporosis."

The alkaline diet tries to prevent this by carefully considering food pH values in an attempt to reduce dietary acid consumption. Although some scientists may disagree, virtually all believe that human existence needs a relatively closely regulated blood pH level of around 7.365–7.4. According to Forbes Magazine, "our bodies go to remarkable lengths to maintain healthy pH levels."

Your pH can fluctuate from 7.35 to 7.45 depending on the time of day, your diet, what you last ate, and when you last used the restroom. If you have electrolyte imbalances and eat too many acidic meals — also known as acid ash foods — your body's fluctuating pH level might lead to greater "acidosis."

What Does "pH Level" Mean?

The word pH relates to the hydrogen potential. It determines the acidity or alkalinity of our body's fluids and tissues.
It is graded on a scale of 0 to 14. The lower the pH of a solution, the more acidic it is. The greater the number, the more alkaline the environment.

A pH of approximately 7 is considered neutral, but because the ideal human body pH is around 7.4, we consider a slightly alkaline pH to be the healthiest.

The body's pH also fluctuates, with the stomach being the most acidic. Even little variations in the pH values of certain species may cause serious problems. For example, as a result of environmental problems such as increased CO_2 deposition, the pH of the ocean has decreased from 8.2 to 8.1, and many ocean life forms have suffered considerably.

The pH level is also essential for plant development, and as a result, it has a significant effect on the mineral content of the meals we consume. Minerals in the ocean, soil and human body serve as pH buffers; thus as acidity increases, mineral levels decrease.

How an Alkaline Diet works

Here is some basic information on acid/alkalinity in the human diet, as well as essential facts regarding how alkaline diets might be beneficial:

When it comes to the overall acid load of the human diet, researchers feel that "there have been significant shifts from hunter-gatherer cultures to the present." Following the agricultural revolution and later extensive industrialization of our food supply over the last 200 years, the food we consume has considerably less potassium, magnesium, and chloride, as well as more salt, than previous diets.

Normally, our kidneys keep our electrolyte levels stable (those of calcium, magnesium, potassium and sodium). When humans are exposed to excessively acidic substances, these electrolytes are employed to neutralize acidity.

According to the previously cited Journal of Environmental Health analysis, the potassium-to-sodium ratio in most people's diets has shifted substantially. The ratio of potassium to sodium used to be 10:1, but it has recently decreased to 1:3. On average, those who follow the "Standard American Diet" ingest three times as much salt as potassium! This substantially helps to an alkaline environment in our bodies.

Many children and adults nowadays consume a high-sodium diet that is deficient in antioxidants, fiber, and critical vitamins, as well as magnesium and potassium. Furthermore, the average Western diet is rich in processed fats, simple carbohydrates, salt, and chloride.

All of these dietary modifications have resulted in an increase in "metabolic acidosis." In other words, many people's bodies' pH levels are no longer appropriate. On top of that, many people have inadequate nutritional intake and issues like potassium and magnesium insufficiency.

Promoting an Alkaline State

Proponents of an alkaline diet argue that contemporary civilization's illnesses, such as cancer and osteoporosis, are caused by consuming a diet with a high acid load. Meats, poultry, dairy, fish, eggs, cereals, and alcohol are all acidic foods. According to some reports, eating too many of these items causes your blood and body fluids to become more acidic.

However, consuming alkaline foods, such as fresh fruit and nuts, causes your blood to become more alkaline, which, according to the diet's supporters, prevents severe health concerns.

A constant pH level, on the other hand, is not typical for your entire body. Your blood pH is about 7.4, but the pH levels in the rest of your body vary significantly. The stomach has a pH of 1.35 to 3.5, which is fairly acidic, and the skin has a pH of 4 to 6.5, according to the Journal of Environmental and Public Health study. Your diet will not affect these closely controlled levels, which exist for a reason;

greater acidity levels, for example, protect the skin from infection and help the stomach to digest food. Some acidity serves a function.

Effects of Alkalinity on Disease

Many proponents of raising blood alkalinity believe that it would prevent chronic diseases such as cancer. According to a comprehensive review published in the June 2016 edition of BMJ Open, no genuine research supports (or refutes) the link between diet acid load and cancer development or therapy.

According to a study published in the Journal of Renal Nutrition in May 2017, an alkaline diet may delay the course of kidney disease or enhance renal function in those who already have it. Your kidneys filter waste, including excess acidity, in order to keep your blood pH around 7.4. A low-acid diet that replaces a large portion of animal protein with plant-based alternatives may be beneficial since your kidneys do not have to work as hard to eliminate the excess acid found in meats, poultry, fish, and dairy.

A high acid diet has been linked to osteoporosis and fast bone loss. To sustain bone density, supporters of a low-acid diet argue that you should maintain alkalinity. In 2019, PEN Nutrition and the Dietitians of Canada published a position paper affirming a lack of data to support the assumption that high-protein (or high-acid) diets increase the dietary acid load, resulting in reduced bone cell development and increased bone loss.

According to research published in Nutrients in April 2018, a normal Western diet with relatively high acid loading would not affect bone mineral density in a statistically significant way for most people. The vast majority of persons have a normal renal function and acid excreting ability. Age, gender, sedentary lifestyle, and race are all risk factors for bone loss. Older individuals with impaired renal function, on the other hand, may benefit from a diet high in alkaline foods. The alkaline diet relieves stress on the kidneys, which are already under stress.

13

Benefits

So, why is an alkaline diet beneficial? Because alkaline meals provide vital nutrients that aid in the prevention of accelerated aging and the progressive loss of organ and cellular functioning. As discussed further below, the benefits of an alkaline diet may include slowing the degradation of tissues and bone density, which can be jeopardized when we are depleted of essential minerals.

1. Protects bone density and muscle mass

Mineral intake is critical for the formation and maintenance of bone structures. According to research, the more alkalizing fruits and vegetables a person consumes, the more protected that person may be against having diminished bone strength and muscle atrophy as they age, a condition known as sarcopenia.

An alkaline diet can benefit bone health by regulating the ratio of minerals necessary for bone formation and mass muscle maintenance, such as calcium, magnesium, and phosphate.

The diet may also aid in the synthesis of growth hormones and vitamin D absorption, which preserves bones while also reducing the risk of many other chronic illnesses.

2. Lowers risk for hypertension and stroke

One of the anti-aging benefits of an alkaline diet is that it reduces inflammation and stimulates growth hormone production. This has been found to boost cardiovascular health and provide protection against common issues such as excessive cholesterol, hypertension (high blood pressure), kidney stones, stroke, and even memory loss.

3. Lowers chronic pain and inflammation

An alkaline diet has been linked to lower levels of chronic pain, according to research. Chronic acidosis has been linked to chronic back pain, migraines, muscle spasms, menstrual irregularities, inflammation, and joint discomfort.

According to one research done by the Society for Minerals and Trace Elements in Germany, when patients with chronic back pain were given an alkaline supplement daily for four weeks, 76 of 82 patients reported substantial pain reductions as assessed by the "Arhus low back pain rating scale."

4. Boosts vitamin absorption and prevents magnesium deficiency

Magnesium is essential for the proper functioning of hundreds of enzyme systems and physiological functions. Many individuals are magnesium deficient, which causes cardiac problems, muscular discomfort, migraines, sleep problems, and anxiety.

Available magnesium is also necessary to activate vitamin D and avoid vitamin D insufficiency, both of which are critical for general immunological and endocrine function.

5. Aids in improving immune function and cancer prevention

When cells lack sufficient minerals to adequately dispose of waste or fully oxygenate the body, the entire body suffers. Mineral loss reduces vitamin absorption, while toxins and infections build in the body and weaken the immune system.

Is it possible that an alkaline diet might help prevent cancer? While the subject is debatable and untested, a study published in the British Journal of Radiology discovered indications that malignant cell death (apoptosis) was more frequent in an alkaline body.

Cancer prevention is thought to be linked to an alkaline shift in pH caused by an adjustment in electric charges and the release of basic protein components. Alkalinity can help reduce inflammation and the risk of illnesses like cancer, and it has been demonstrated that an alkaline diet is more helpful for some chemotherapeutic drugs that require a higher pH to operate properly.

6. Can assist you in maintaining your healthy weight

Although the diet isn't primarily focused on fat loss, sticking to an alkaline diet meal plan for weight loss can assist guard against obesity.

Limiting acid-forming meals and increasing alkaline-forming foods may make losing weight easier owing to the diet's capacity to lower leptin levels and inflammation. This has an impact on both your appetite and your ability to burn fat.

Because alkaline-forming foods are anti-inflammatory, following an alkaline diet allows your body to attain normal leptin levels and feel satiated with eating the number of calories it requires.

7. It will make your skin glow

Whether you have acne, rosacea, eczema, psoriasis, or aged skin, there is one thing in common: ALL skin issues are ACID problems! Your skin is the body's biggest organ and the "third kidney," serving as a vital organ for detoxification.

Urination, feces, respiration, and perspiration are the four primary detoxification processes. If you notice ANYTHING on your skin, it's an indication that you're acidic and your body is working hard to get these acids out. When you see the signs and symptoms on your skin, it's time to alkalize.

Whatever the problem is with your skin, chances are it starts and ends with what you consume, and sugar and wheat are the main offenders. I recommend reducing or completely removing them from your diet.

14

The Acne Diet: Eating to Cause Clear Skin

Do you want to know how to get rid of acne? The so-called acne diet might be a good place to start. But, before we get into the formula for an acne-free diet, let's go over the fundamentals.

1. What is acne?

Acne is a skin disorder that occurs when pores get blocked with debris, oil, or bacteria, resulting in irritation.

2. What causes acne?

Acne is caused by a variety of causes, but the major culprits appear to be excess sebum, hormones, and germs.

3. How diet and acne are related?

What you consume has an impact on how your body operates as a whole. So it goes to reason that what is excellent for acne is similar to what is good for a healthy body in general.

The Acne Diet

Recent diet and acne research have revealed that a low-sugar, well-balanced diet is optimal for decreasing inflammation and controlling hormone (and hence, sebum) levels.

Here are our top diet suggestions for clean skin:

Drink more water

Staying hydrated is a matter of nutrition 101. After all, your body is composed of 60% water. Therefore it should come as no surprise that you need to drink adequate water to improve bodily functions. Drinking water is also important for eating the proper number of daily calories - we frequently confuse hunger with thirst, so when in doubt, drink water first. Water is the basis of good, clean skin, so drink at least 8 glasses each day.

Cut back on sugar

Sugar is categorically not allowed in any acne diet. Unfortunately, it is present in almost everything we eat during the day, making it impossible to avoid. Limit your daily sugar consumption to two to four servings of fructose found in fruit, and avoid sugars found elsewhere, such as processed carbs and candy aisle sweets. Sugar, especially from specific sources, can aggravate acne and create a slew of other health issues.

Cut back on alcohol

Most alcoholic beverages are extremely sweet and hence unhealthy. Then there's the basic and stark reality that alcohol is a toxin you choose to put in your body (and presumably pay a lot of money for) that may cause heart disease, stroke, and dementia, to name a few terrible side-effects. Forget about your skin — almost every organ in your body despises alcohol. It, if you do drink, do so in moderation – and drink enough water to offset the effects of alcohol.

Avoid processed foods

Processed foods include more sugars, salts, and fats than we need, but meals prepared at home with fresh ingredients are healthier since you can regulate what goes into them. It may appear complicated and pricey at first, but after you've equipped your kitchen with the essential culinary materials you need on a regular basis, you'll discover that cooking at home is not only healthier but also less expensive. You'll never eat anything from a box again.

Ditch dairy (but keep Greek yogurt)

Dairy has a lot of sugar (yes, lactose is also a sugar, just like glucose and fructose). However, dairy consumption has been related to an increase in acne. Although dairy is abundant in minerals our systems want, such as calcium and protein, animal-based protein may not be the best source of protein since research after study has connected animal-based proteins to an increased risk of cancer.

The research isn't completely definitive, so you don't have to give up meat and cheese forever, but physicians increasingly believe that reducing your consumption of animal proteins in favor of more veggies is a smart idea, both for your skin and for your overall health.

You don't have to eliminate dairy entirely: as a source of calcium, protein, and probiotics, try a sugar-free (or as near to sugar-free as possible) Greek yogurt.

Ingredients to include on your menu as soon as possible

Vegetables with green leaves

Recent fad diets, such as the alkaline diet, called for balancing your body's pH by eating more "alkaline" foods and eating less "acidic" ones.

The fact is that our bodies already manage our internal pH, but that doesn't mean that this diet fad, which promotes eating vegetables, isn't on to something. Supporters suggest beets, broccoli, cauliflower, celery, cucumber, kale, lettuce, onions, peas, peppers, and spinach. It's hardly rocket science: the more veggies you eat, the clearer your skin will be and the healthier your body will be. The acne diet is the way to go.

Antioxidant-rich berries
The more antioxidants you can eat, such as veggies, the better — especially if you suffer from acne. A high-antioxidant diet can help reduce mild to severe acne. That's why berries are so tasty — try blueberries, blackberries, cherries, and goji berries.

Dark chocolate
The healthiest kind of chocolate is dark chocolate. (It's low in sugar and, depending on the kind, has very little to no dairy.) It also includes zinc, which is an anti-acne vitamin. Fortunately, it's also tasty, so go ahead and indulge (in moderation, of course).

Oysters
Oysters are well-known aphrodisiacs, but their zinc concentration is quite high, so depending on what you're seeking, oysters can satisfy all of your demands in a single meal (wink). Just be sure your oysters are grown in a sustainable manner.

Pumpkin seeds
Not a fan of shellfish? No need to worry; zinc may be found in a variety of different locations. Sprinkle some pumpkin seeds on top of a salad for a daily dose of zinc, or eat them as a snack at work.

Green Tea

Green tea is high in polyphenols (poly-what?), so try integrating it into your diet. Don't be concerned about how to pronounce them; just know that polyphenols improve blood flow and oxygen to the skin, enhancing its general appearance, feel, and, most importantly, health.

15

Seven-Day Alkaline Diet Plan to Rebalance PH Levels and Fight Inflammation

The importance of PH balance in human health cannot be overstated. It is an abbreviation for the power of hydrogen, which is a measurement of the concentration of hydrogen ions in the body. The pH scale goes from 1 to 14, with 7 being considered neutral. Solutions with a pH less than 7 are considered to be acidic, whereas those with a pH of more than 7 are said to be basic or alkaline. Our optimum pH range is somewhat alkaline, ranging from 7.30 to 7.45. You may check your pH levels on a regular basis by dipping a litmus paper into your saliva or urine first thing in the morning before eating or drinking anything.

An alkaline diet is required to restore PH levels. Because it excludes acidic foods that promote inflammation and disease, this diet is an excellent choice for those looking to restore their PH levels and fight inflammation. Bloating, sleeplessness, poor memory, kidney stones, low energy levels, high blood pressure, migraines, diabetes, heart disease, muscular discomfort, and weak bones are all prevented by alkaline diets.

Furthermore, alkaline diets aid in weight reduction and the treatment of arthritis, inflammation, and cancer! They raise blood acidity, and the body leeches minerals from bones and organs to restore the appropriate pH balance of 7.4. The PH levels are also crucial for cell signaling, which is required for your cells to fulfill their specific functions.

I'd like to share with you a 7-day alkaline food plan to help you restore your PH levels and reduce inflammation. Vicki Edgson, a nutritional therapist, and Natasha Corrett, an organic chef, are the designers of this alkaline diet plan. This diet's objective is to keep the pH between 7.35 and 7.45. This may be accomplished by eating 80 percent alkaline and 20 percent acidic meals.

You should eat foods like vegetables, fruits, peas, legumes, beans, soybeans, tofu, almonds, seeds, olive oil, coconut oil, and flaxseed oil if you follow an alkaline diet plan. There is also a list of foods that must be ingested, such as artichoke, asparagus, broccoli, beetroot, dates, figs, cauliflower, fennel, lemon, kale, spinach, and watercress.

You should also restrict your consumption of processed meals. Sugar, dairy, meat, eggs, alcohol, most cereals, caffeine, soy, processed maize, safflower and sunflower oils, hydrogenated oil, and margarine.

Here is a 7-day alkaline diet plan:

Day 1
Breakfast: chia and strawberry quinoa
Snack: an orange
Lunch: sweet and savory salad
Snack: 1/2 cup toasted nuts and dried fruits
Dinner: Roasted chicken (3-4 oz.) with roasted sweet potatoes and parsnips, simple green salad with olive oil and apple cider vinegar

Day 2
Breakfast: vegan apple parfait
Snack: 1 pear
Lunch: white bean stew with savory avocado wraps
Snack: One handful of toasted pumpkin seeds

Dinner: Salad of cucumbers with olive oil and apple cider vinegar Roasted chicken (3-4 oz.) with roasted Brussels sprouts and red peppers

Day 3
Breakfast: purple berry smoothie
Snack: 1 mango
Lunch: Asian sesame dressing and noodles
Snack: a handful of dried apricot
Dinner: 4 oz. cooked fish, 1/2 baked sweet potato, curried beets, and greens

Day 4
Breakfast: apple and almond butter oats
Snack: 1 banana
Lunch: green goddess bowl
Snack: a handful of almonds
Dinner: kale pesto zucchini noodles

Day 5
Breakfast: power smoothie
Snack: an avocado
Lunch: quinoa burrito bowl
Snack: a handful of dates
Dinner: wild rice mushroom and almond risotto

Day 6
Breakfast: chia breakfast pudding
Snack: 1/2 cup blueberries
Lunch: miso soup with fermented tofu
Snack: a handful of macadamia nuts
Dinner: roasted root vegetables with 4 oz salmon

Day 7
Breakfast: quinoa porridge
Snack: A few slices of cantaloupe
Lunch: Mexican quinoa salad
Snack: A handful of coconut slices that have been dried
Dinner: pumpkin soup

16

Apple Cider Vinegar for Acne

Among the several at-home DIY skincare treatments available, employing apple cider vinegar to help clear up acne is one of the most well-known—and contentious. Some swear by it on the internet, but others (including many dermatologists) warn that it may be too stripping, especially when taken undiluted.

What are the skin clearing benefits of apple cider vinegar?

For some skin types, an at-home apple cider vinegar toner may be effective in exfoliating and preventing acne. Others, though, may find it ineffective—and if not diluted, it may cause discomfort. Unfiltered apple cider vinegar is favored for skincare and many other health-boosting applications (both internally and topically, such as on the hair and scalp). This is due to the presence of the "mother," or the murky, brown-tinged strands of bacteria and enzymes that are considered to be the source of many of the elixir's benefits, in unfiltered apple cider vinegar. While no studies on apple cider vinegar and acne have been conducted, ACV does contain numerous research-backed characteristics that may be responsible for its reported capacity to help control breakouts.

1. It may help balance the skin's pH.

If you've ever drunk or smelled apple cider vinegar, you'll notice straight once that it's acidic—very acidic. ACV has a pH between 2 and 3 on a scale of 0 (acidic) to 14 (alkaline). Healthy skin with a strong and intact barrier is also somewhat acidic, with an optimal pH level of 5.5, whereas damaged skin barriers (particularly those with skin problems like eczema and rosacea) have a higher, more alkaline pH level. So it seems to reason that using apple cider vinegar to the skin might help restore its natural, slightly acidic pH levels—but other doctors and research studies disagree. "The lower pH of ACV has been found to help regulate the skin pH and enhance skin barrier function in diseases like atopic dermatitis, where the pH is more alkaline," says holistic board-certified dermatologist Keira Barr, M.D. "However, [some] research contradict it."

2. Acts as a chemical exfoliant.

Apple cider vinegar is also a powerful chemical exfoliator. It's naturally high in alpha-hydroxy acids (AHAs), which are the same chemicals found in our favorite toners and face peels to help slough off dead skin. According to Barr, ACV includes "alpha-hydroxy acids such as lactic, citric, and malic acids." These acids, when applied topically, "exfoliate the topmost layers of the skin, revealing skin that appears smoother and more moisturized." As previously stated, utilizing chemical exfoliants on a daily basis can help level out and smooth skin tone, thereby decreasing the appearance of acne scars. While this may be true anecdotally and theoretically, Barr points out that there is presently no strong scientific research to support ACV's acne-scar-fading properties.

3. It has antifungal and antibacterial properties.

Aside from exfoliating, these natural AHAs are multifunctional; acetic acid, for example, "has antifungal and antibacterial characteristics that may help kill the bacteria that causes acne," according to Barr. Citric acid and lactic acid have also been found in studies to destroy Cutibacterium acnes (previously known as Propionibacterium acnes, or P. acnes), a kind of bacteria on the skin that has been linked to the development of acne.

Instructions on how to make apple cider vinegar toner at home:

1. Combine the apple cider vinegar and water in a mixing bowl.

When used as a DIY toner, apple cider vinegar must be diluted. Because it is so acidic, "if not adequately diluted, ACV can cause superficial chemical burns and skin irritation," says board-certified dermatologist Dhaval Bhanusali, M.D.

Make a solution of one part vinegar to three or four parts water (for sensitive skin types, even more water). Furthermore, "before applying it on your face for the first time, try a test area on your skin to ensure you won't have an unpleasant response," Barr advises.

- For severe acne, use one part apple cider vinegar to three parts water.
- For moderate acne, use one part apple cider vinegar to four parts water.
- For sensitive skin, dilute 1 part apple cider vinegar to 5 parts water.

Because this homemade toner will not include the same stabilizers or preservatives as store-bought alternatives, it must be produced fresh before use. Mix each single-use dosage in a shot glass to avoid wasting ACV.

2. As tolerated, apply to skin.

Apply a cotton ball or reusable cloth pads to clean skin to apply this diluted apple cider vinegar and water combination like a toner. Begin slowly and gently; apply a small amount of toner to the skin and leave it on for a few minutes before rinsing. If it's well-tolerated, Barr recommends increasing the amount of toner used or the length of time it's left on the face—but never leave ACV on your skin for more than 15 minutes. After thoroughly washing, add a moisturizer. Barr suggests using ACV toner once or twice a week, as tolerated.

3. It may be used as spot therapy.

If you simply want to target a few regions of your face, such as your chin, T-zone, or even a single zit, you may not need to use the toner on your whole face. The same guidelines apply when used as a spot treatment; simply limit your application regions. This will aid in the drying of particular blemishes without the need to treat the whole face.

Who shouldn't use it:

Using an apple cider vinegar toner on naturally dry skin may be too drying. If you have an open wound, such as pimples or pustules that have come to a head (or been popped), using apple cider vinegar topically may hurt. If you have very sensitive or acne-prone skin, your skin barrier is typically weakened. Therefore it's always a good idea to see a dermatologist before putting any DIY concoctions to your face, ACV or otherwise. "Applying ACV straight to the skin, especially for those with really sensitive skin, maybe quite harmful," Barr adds. "When used at maximum dosage on the skin, there is a danger of producing redness, irritation, and serious chemical burns."

Conclusion

Pores are small openings in your skin that may get clogged by oil, germs, dead skin cells, and debris. When this happens, you may get a pimple or a "zit." If this problem affects your skin on a regular basis, you may have acne.

Acne is the most prevalent skin ailment in the United States, according to the American Academy of Dermatology. Although acne is not a life-threatening illness, it may be excruciatingly uncomfortable, especially when severe. It can also induce mental anguish.

Acne on your face can lower your self-esteem and, in the long run, create lasting physical scars.

Acne prevention is challenging. However, there are actions you may take at home to help avoid acne following therapy.

These stages are as follows:
- Using an oil-free cleanser twice a day on your face.
- Removing extra oil with an over-the-counter acne cream
- Staying away from oil-based cosmetics.
- You are thoroughly cleansing your skin and removing makeup before going to bed.
- I was showering after working out.
- I am avoiding apparel that is too tight.
- It is consuming a nutritious diet that is low in processed sugars.
- Lowering stress

Made in the USA
Middletown, DE
11 January 2024

47682606R00060